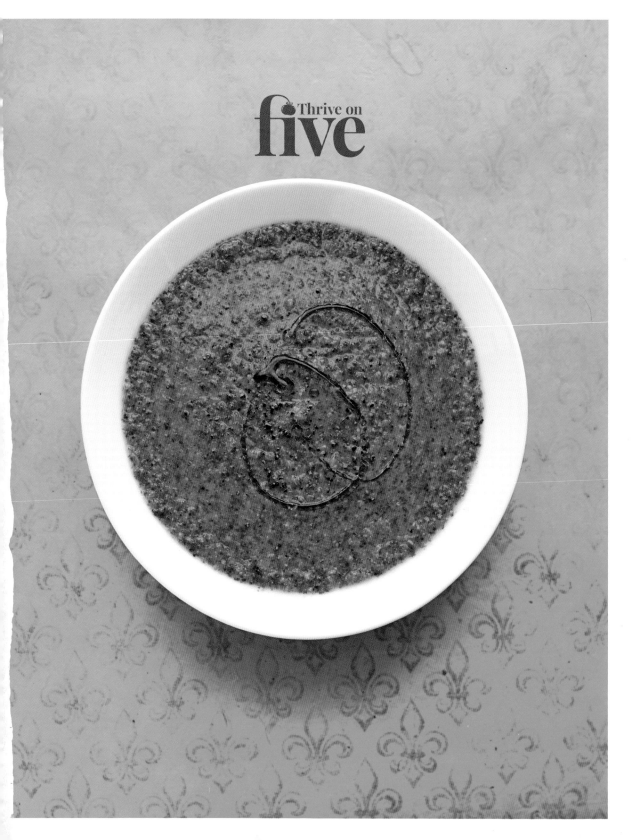

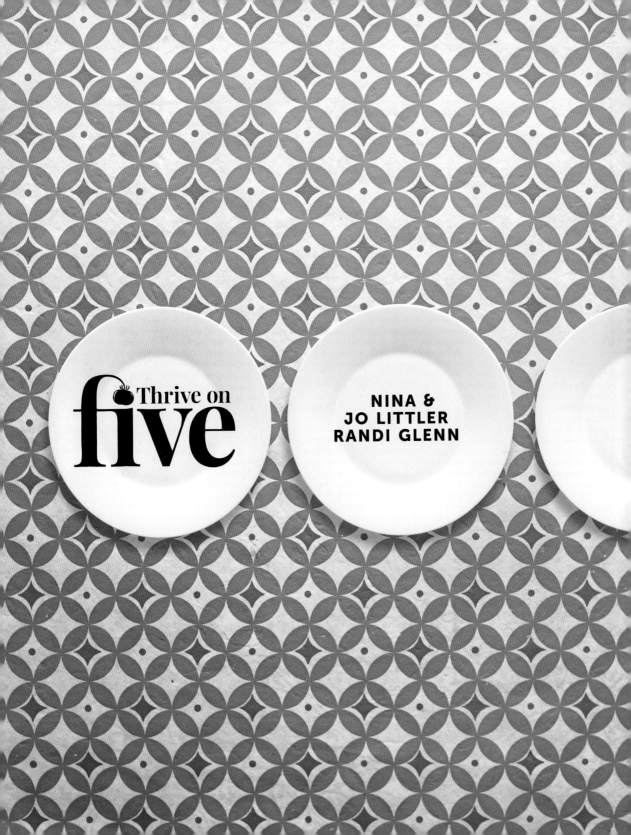

Thrive on five

NINA & JO LITTLER RANDI GLENN

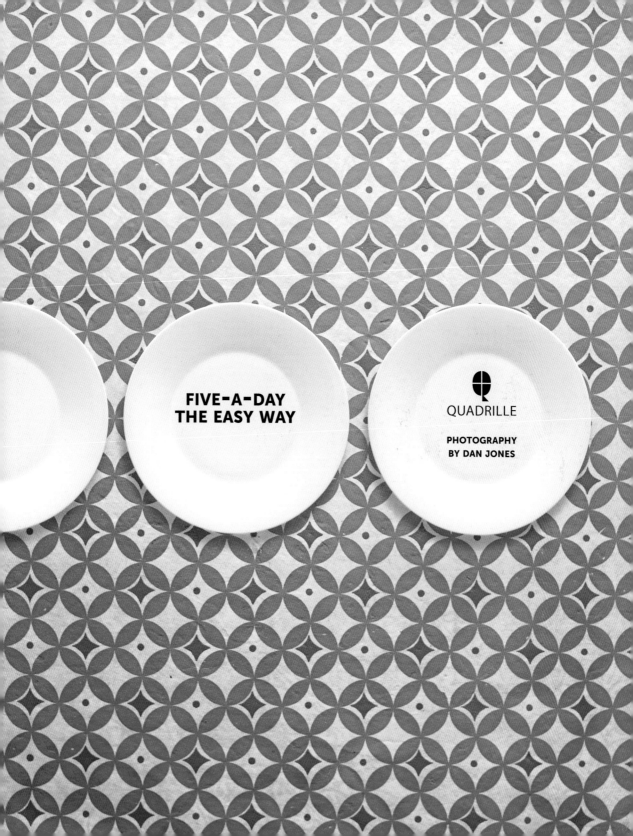

**FIVE-A-DAY
THE EASY WAY**

QUADRILLE

**PHOTOGRAPHY
BY DAN JONES**

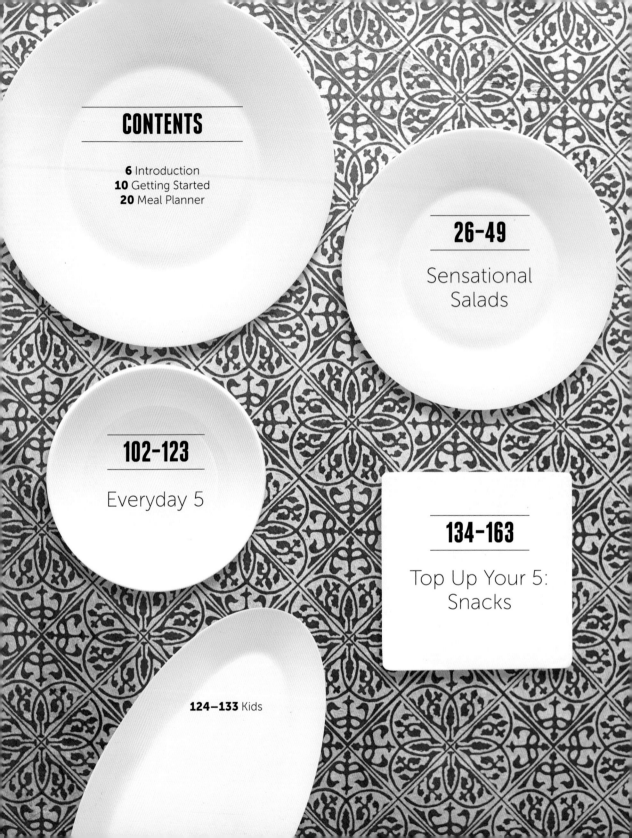

CONTENTS

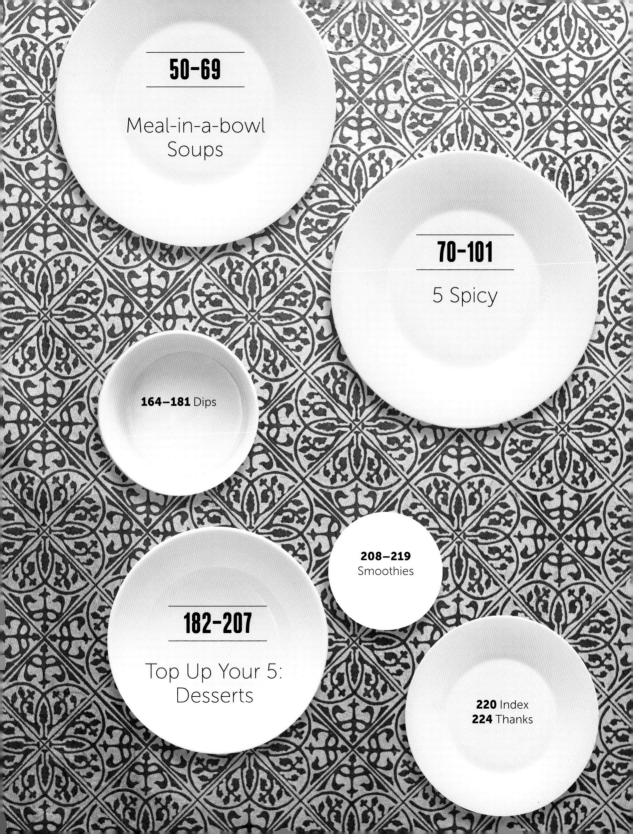

THRIVE ON FIVE
FIVE-A-DAY THE EASY WAY

Many of us think we get our five portions of fruit and veg a day regularly... but most of us actually fall short, with even 'healthy' eaters often underestimating what they need. Did you know, for instance, that most shop-bought salads contain only one or two portions? Despite our efforts, the average intake is still only 3.5 portions a day. And this is in the face of growing evidence which suggests that five-a-day should be a minimum target, with increasing numbers of countries issuing guidelines for their citizens to eat five portions of vegetables plus two of fruits daily, or seven portions, or ten portions, or even vegetables 'in abundance', for optimum health. It's clear that more is – in this case – better.

But don't worry. This book will make it really easy to eat at least five-a-day. Taking inspiration from around the world, most of our recipes contain all of your five-a-day, while others will help you add extra portions through snacks, puddings or drinks. Ensuring you get your five-a-day in a tasty way has never been easier, we have done all the work for you. All you need to do now is to make the food! And we've even made that simple: all the recipes have easy-to-find ingredients and none are hard to cook. If you eat one of our five-a-day dishes for lunch, then the job's done and you've no need to worry about how much fruit and veg you eat in the evening. If you pick up a piece of fruit or eat more veg in the rest of the day, you'll exceed the goal.

HOW OFTEN ARE YOU EATING YOUR FIVE-A-DAY?

WHY FIVE?

The five-a-day idea was conceived in California in 1991 at the National Cancer Institute, then adopted by the World Health Organisation in 2003. Its influence grew rapidly, spreading around the globe, and it is now a near-universal concept.

We all need to eat more fruits and vegetables, particularly vegetables, as they are lower in sugars. The proven health benefits are enormous: reduced risk of heart disease, strokes, obesity, type-2 diabetes and some cancers. Eating more vegetables allows us to maintain a healthier weight, helps reduce cholesterol and gives us better resistance to common ailments such as colds. To take full advantage of the wide variety of phytochemicals and nutrients in fruits and vegetables, we should ideally eat at least five portions of five different types each day. Our recipes are designed to help you do just that.

Fruits and vegetables should make up about one-third of our daily food, according to NHS guidelines. These foods are not only high in fibre and low in fat, they are also a rich source of vitamins, minerals and other health-giving substances such as antioxidants, essential for good health and protection against all kinds of disease.

THE CHALLENGE

The five-a-day message is drummed into us daily – by the media, at the doctor's surgery, or as we wander down the supermarket aisle – but we still fall short of the target. Why? It's not that we lack good intentions. In fact in the most recent recorded year we threw away more than 12 billion portions of fruits and vegetables!

Research tells us there are two simple reasons. First, preparing vegetables that the family all like with every meal can be time-consuming. Second, most of us just don't find vegetables interesting enough. But with the range of new, creative recipe ideas in this book, vegetables never need to be a plain or boring afterthought again.

Making vegetables really tasty and easy to prepare is the key to meeting the five-a-day challenge and we believe, with this collection of recipes, that we've done it. As you become a regular Thrive on Five cook, you'll probably find you are naturally eating meat less often. You don't need it with every meal but, for those days when it is on the menu, we have suggested which recipes go well with meat, or indeed fish.

OUR RECIPES AND YOUR LIFESTYLE

Whether you're vegetarian, vegan, dairy-free, gluten-free or low-carb, you'll find plenty of dishes here to suit you. And most of them can easily be adapted for other diets. Many of our recipes are already low in calories but, if your goal is to lose weight, you can reduce the calorie count further by limiting the amount of oil or cheese you use.

And there's no denying that snacking is now part of everyday life, but the most common snacks – think crisps and biscuits – are not always healthy. If you're in the mood to snack, we have added a section of tempting recipes which include anything from one to four portions of veg, to use as a 'top up' to help you get to five-a-day.

One beauty of so many of our dishes is that you can make them in larger quantities and store them in the fridge so, when you get in late from work or don't have time to cook for the kids, there's no need to microwave a ready-meal or head for the take-away. Instead, you can eat a delicious, hearty meal that is also doing you all good.

WHAT IS A PORTION, AND HOW TO USE THIS BOOK

Adults should eat at least five 80g portions of five different fruits or vegetables a day. Many people don't realise, for example, that even if you're mad on broccoli and eat it until it comes out of your ears, it still only counts as one portion. Our recipes use more convenient measures where possible but we also include the intended gram weight of the relevant ingredients, so it's easy to see where your portions are coming from.

Children should aim for five different varieties of fruits or vegetables a day but they need not eat the full 80g of each. Our Kids 5 recipes are based on five portions of 40g each, while most of our Everyday 5 recipes are intended to serve two adults and two children.

Smoothies which include two or more whole vegetables or fruits only count as two of your five-a-day, however much you put in.

Beans and pulses count as only one of your five-a-day, however much you eat.

Potatoes do not count (but sweet potatoes do).

For a fuller description of what counts as a portion, the government produces a guide that can be found at www.nhs.uk/Livewell/5ADAY/Documents/Downloads/5ADAY_portion_guide.pdf

GETTING STARTED: EAT THE RAINBOW

Colour is an excellent indicator of the different nutrients in fresh fruits and vegetables. Each shade offers a unique benefit to our health. So don't just eat your greens, eat your oranges, reds, purples and whites, too!

ORANGE/YELLOW

Carotenoids give orange/ yellow vegetables and fruits their colour. Beta-carotene – found in carrots, sweet potatoes, pumpkins and mangos – is a particularly important carotenoid. It is used to produce vitamin A, which helps maintain healthy skin, eyes and immune systems. Orange and yellow citrus fruits are very good sources of vitamin C.

RED

The red colour of many fruits and vegetables – tomatoes or watermelons, for example – is due to the plant pigment lycopene. This is a powerful antioxidant which has been shown to limit damage to cells and help reduce the risk of heart disease and some cancers, particularly prostate cancer. Lycopene has also been shown to prevent damage caused by sun exposure. Most red fruits and vegetables are also rich sources of vitamin C.

BLUE/PURPLE

Anthocyanin is the plant pigment which gives blue/purple – and some red – vegetables and fruits their colour. Think of beetroots, blackberries and blueberries. Anthocyanins have strong antioxidant properties, which have been shown to reduce the risk of cell damage, some cancers, heart disease and strokes.

GREEN

Green fruits and vegetables get their colour from the plant pigment chlorophyll, and they contain a range of phytochemicals which have been shown to have anti-cancer properties. Green leafy vegetables are also an excellent source of folate, iron and vitamin C, which in turn helps the absorption of iron.

WHITE

White or white/yellow fruits and vegetables get their colour from a compound called anthoxanthin, which may lower the risk of heart disease and help to relieve the pain and swelling of arthritis. Some white produce, such as garlic, contains allicin which has antibacterial and antiviral properties and may help reduce high blood pressure and high cholesterol.

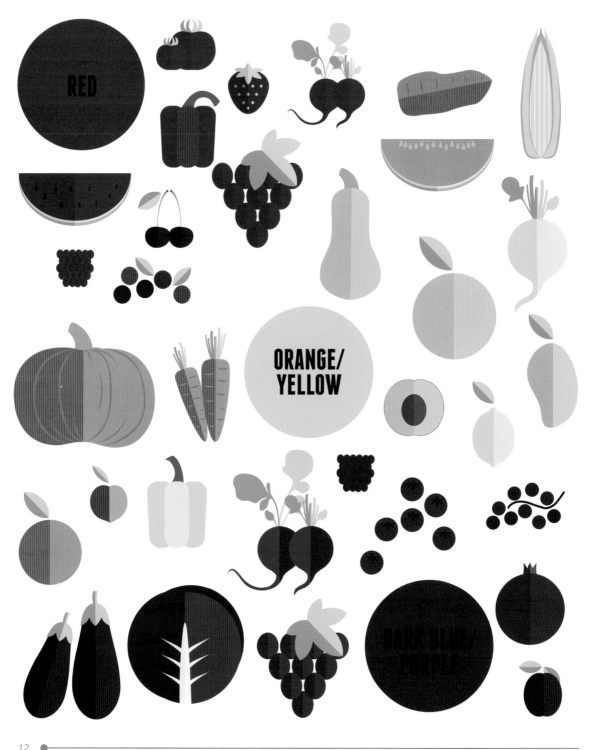

RED

ORANGE/
YELLOW

DARK BLUE/
PURPLE

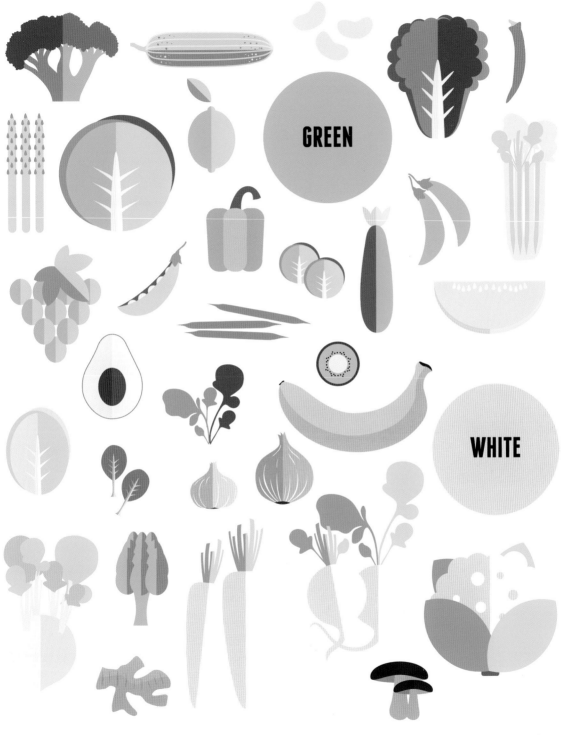

GREEN

WHITE

ROOT-TO-FLOWER EATING

Including all the different parts of plants in our diet not only gives us a variety of nutrients, but also offers a whole host of contrasting textures, which make vegetable dishes much more interesting to eat. Vegetables and fruits can be derived from many parts of a plant, including those fruits that often masquerade as vegetables, such as avocados, aubergines, cucumbers, peppers, squashes and tomatoes.

Vegetables that grow above ground – with the exception of seeds and pulses – can usually be eaten raw or require light cooking only, for example steaming, microwaving, stir-frying or light roasting.

Vegetables that grow below ground can usually withstand higher cooking temperatures and need longer to cook. Suitable cooking methods include roasting or longer simmering.

BELOW GROUND:

Roots: *beetroot, carrot, celeriac, parsnip, radish, swede, turnip*

Bulbs and tubers: *garlic, leek, onion, shallot, spring onion, sweet potato*

ABOVE GROUND:

Stems and shoots: *asparagus, bamboo shoot, celery, fennel, kohlrabi*

Leaves: *cabbage, kale, lettuce, pak choi, spinach, watercress*

Flowers: *artichoke, broccoli, cauliflower*

Fruits: *aubergine, avocado, cucumber, okra, pepper, pumpkin, squash, tomato*

Seeds: *corn, peas*

Pulses: *beans, chickpeas, lentils*

COOK CAREFULLY

Most fruits and many vegetables can be eaten raw, which maintains their nutritional value. But some are even more nutritious when lightly cooked, as cooking helps release their nutrients, for example lycopene from tomatoes and beta-carotene from peppers. Cooking helps release starch and other nutritional substances from some vegetables, making it easier for our bodies to use them.

Steaming and blanching vegetables is a much better cooking method than boiling. Heat destroys nutrients and they can leak into cooking water. So it is best to limit the amount of water you use and the time you leave your vegetables simmering.

Oven roasting, either with a little oil or dry roasting without oil, really concentrates the flavours of vegetables. It will caramelise those that can withstand higher cooking temperatures and require a longer cooking time, such as root vegetables and tubers.

Roasting vegetables with or without oil is also a great way to cook lots of vegetables at once and perfect for aubergines, carrots, courgettes, mushrooms, onions, peppers and squashes. Once roasted, you're much more likely to eat them.

Lightly stir-frying is a good way to cook vegetables quickly, but restrict the amount of oil you use to keep the fat content down. If you stir-fry, avoid using olive oil as it breaks down at higher temperatures (save it for salads, or for dressing raw vegetables). Sunflower oil is a good substitute.

Microwaving chopped vegetables in a little water is an excellent and quick way to cook them. Frozen vegetables and pre-washed leaves such as spinach cook very well in their plastic packaging.

Save deep-fried vegetables for an occasional treat.

STORE SENSIBLY

Cutting vegetables, thus exposing them to light and oxygen, causes damage which can destroy nutrients, so it is best to chop vegetables just before cooking. If you do pre-prepare, seal and store fresh chopped vegetables in the fridge, in the dark, to prolong their life.

Most green vegetables store well in the fridge.

Potatoes, sweet potatoes and onions should be kept in a cool, dark place. Don't keep potatoes in the fridge, as they will lose some of their taste.

Avoid plastic bags where possible, as these do not let the vegetables breathe and allow moisture to build up. Paper bags are better.

Keep vegetables that are past their best away from fresh vegetables, as keeping them together accelerates decomposition.

Use up leftover carrot, onion and celery to make stock. (You can portion this up and freeze it.)

Corn on the cob freezes well without pre-cooking. From frozen, simply boil for eight minutes and it will taste like fresh corn.

We do not recommend freezing French beans or peas. The commercial methods used for freezing these create a superior frozen product. Beans and peas tend to lose their colour and texture when frozen at home.

If you have a glut of tomatoes, it is best to blanch and skin them (see page 180) before freezing. Or make a sauce by skinning tomatoes, then cooking them for 40 minutes to one hour. You can portion this up in bags and freeze. Add chilli if you prefer a spiced tomato sauce.

Cook fresh vegetables that are starting to look tired, then store them in the fridge. This will buy you more time, so you have longer to eat them.

TOPPING-UP TIPS

Buy your favourite vegetables and fruits when they are in season, cook them and freeze them, and you will have a ready supply. Butternut squash, corn, courgette and pumpkin can be chopped and frozen without pre-cooking; just add straight from the freezer to a soup, curry or stew.

When making soups, curries or stews, add a couple of handfuls of spinach or other greens towards the end of the cooking time.

One heaped tablespoon of tomato purée counts as one of your five-a-day and is really easy to add to a variety of dishes.

Add 'meaty' pulses such as lentils or borlotti or pinto beans to dishes such as chilli or lasagne. The canned varieties are particularly convenient.

Blitzing onion, celery and carrot finely and adding to the base of a soup, curry, stew or bake provides extra portions of vegetables, adds great flavour and reduces the need for stock powder.

Salad leaves are nutritious but they are very light, so for one 80g portion you need a large bowlful. But watercress and herbs count too and they will add flavour and interest to your salad leaves.

Even breakfast is a great time to start thinking about five-a-day. A traditional English cooked breakfast can get you there. Beans, tomatoes and mushrooms with a glass of juice will give you four of your five portions. Then try adding a portion of spinach – great with eggs – and you'll get to five!

Make any of our delicious dips (see pages 164–181) and leave them in the fridge. If you need a quick snack, or if the kids are hungry after school, you'll be amazed at how quickly dips get devoured. If raw vegetables are ready-chopped for use as dippers, these usually disappear quickly, too...

EVEN BREAKFAST IS A GREAT TIME TO START THINKING ABOUT FIVE-A-DAY

THIS 14-DAY PLANNER WILL HELP GET YOU STARTED COOKING THE THRIVE ON FIVE WAY

We've suggested a number of combinations here which will give you the flexibility to pick five, seven or even more, depending on your particular lifestyle and how many portions you are aiming for. Each day you will get a wide variety of vegetables as well as some fruits, with the occasional treat thrown in.

The meals suggested here are not supposed to be your total food intake for one day, just the fruit and veg part. But whatever else you choose for your other meals and snacks, you'll know you're already quids in where your five-a-day are concerned.

DAY ONE

Breakfast/pudding: Summer berry compôte with Greek yogurt **+2**

Lunch: Broccoli, fennel and Stilton soup **+5**

Dip: Chunky courgette, pepper and chilli salsa **+3**

TOTAL: **+10**

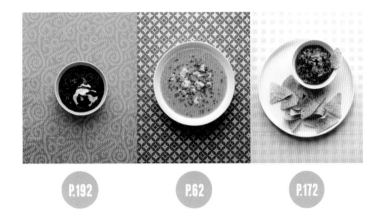

P.192   P.62   P.172

DAY TWO

Lunch: Courgette, carrot and feta fritters **+2**

Light supper: Peanut spiced vegetables **+5**

Snack: Raisin and apricot flapjack **+1**

TOTAL: **+8**

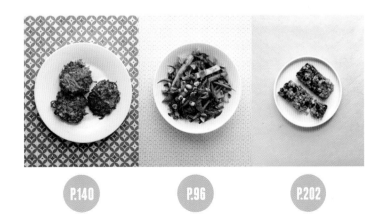

P.140   P.96   P.202

DAY THREE

Breakfast/snack: Avocado, banana and raspberry energiser **+2**

Lunch: Herby stuffed mushrooms **+2**

Dinner: Pisto con huevos **+5**

TOTAL: **+9**

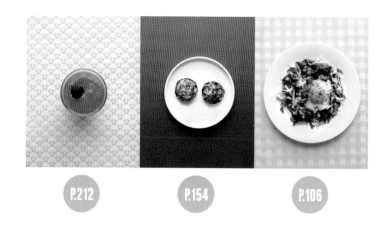

P.212   P.154   P.106

DAY FOUR

Dip: Gorgeous guacamole **+2**

Dinner: Smoky chipotle chilli **+5**

Pudding: Exotic Eton mess **+2**

TOTAL: **+9**

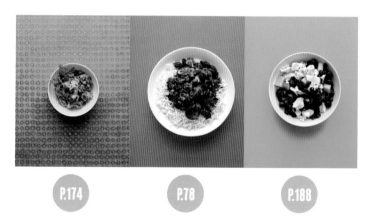

P.174   P.78   P.188

DAY FIVE

Breakfast/snack: Carrot, apple and ginger juice **+2**

Lunch: Minted green garden soup **+5**

Dinner: Thrive on Five's famous pasty **+3**

TOTAL: **+10**

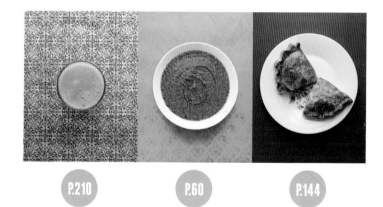

P.210   P.60   P.144

DAY SIX

Breakfast/snack: Watermelon, strawberry and mint crush **+2**

Lunch: 'Tabbouleh' with lentils, red grapes and feta **+5**

Light supper: Sweet potato and courgette falafel **+2**

TOTAL: **+9**

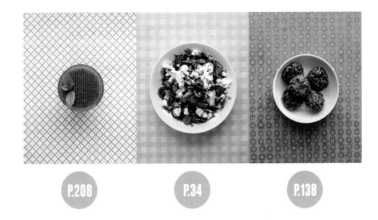

P.208 P.34 P.138

DAY SEVEN

Breakfast/snack: Spiced carrot and date muffin **+2**

Lunch: Minted pea and pepper nori **+2**

Dinner: Tangy fennel and artichoke salad with olives and caper berries **+5**

TOTAL: **+9**

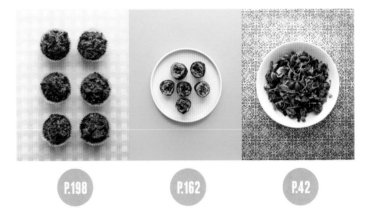

P.198 P.162 P.42

DAY EIGHT

Dip: Tomato, avocado and mango salsa **+2**

Lunch: Roast Med veg wrap **+4**

Dinner: Fragrant cauliflower soup with coconut and lemon grass **+5**

TOTAL: **+11**

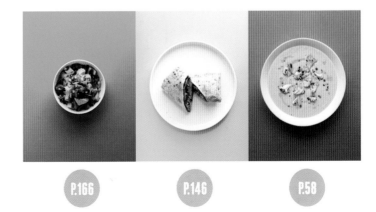

P.166 P.146 P.58

DAY NINE

Breakfast/snack: Melon, cucumber and lime zinger **+2**

Dip: Baba ghanoush **+2**

Dinner: Fruity quinoa salad **+5**

TOTAL: **+9**

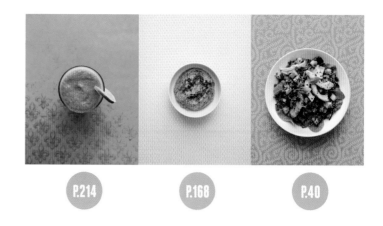

P.214   P.168   P.40

DAY TEN

Breakfast/snack: Blood orange, pumpkin and flaxseed smoothie **+2**

Lunch: Courgette frittata **+2**

Light supper: Warm roasted roots with buffalo mozzarella and balsamic **+5**

TOTAL: **+9**

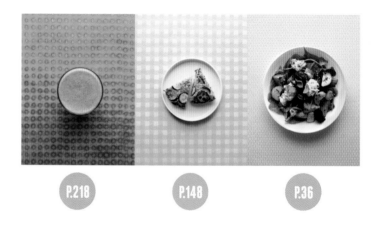

P.218   P.148   P.36

DAY ELEVEN

Dip: Cucumber and banana raita **+1**

Dinner: Pligouri **+5**

Pudding: Chocolate and orange chickpea mousse **+2**

TOTAL: **+8**

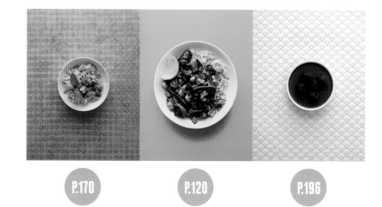

P.170   P.120   P.196

DAY TWELVE

Lunch: Cucumber and houmous maki **+2**

Snack: Pineapple loaf with flaxseed **+1**

Dinner: Thai green curry **+5**

TOTAL: **+8**

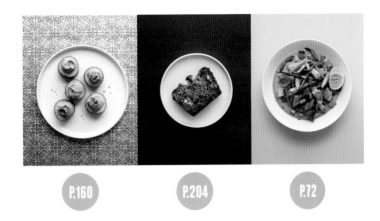

P.160   P.204   P.72

DAY THIRTEEN

Breakfast/snack: Apple, blackberry and beetroot refresher **+2**

Dip: Carrot tzatziki **+1**

Dinner: Goan aubergine curry with coconut and tamarind **+5**

TOTAL: **+8**

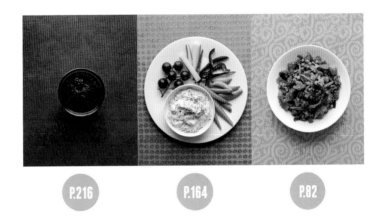

P.216   P.164   P.82

DAY FOURTEEN

Lunch: Spiced involtini primavera **+2**

Dinner: Stir-fried oriental noodles with ginger and sesame **+5**

Pudding: Rhubarb and strawberry sorbet with ginger cream **+2**

TOTAL: **+9**

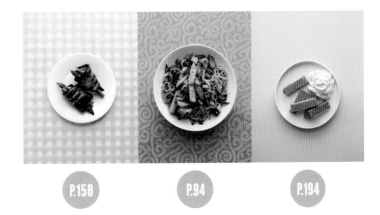

P.158   P.94   P.194

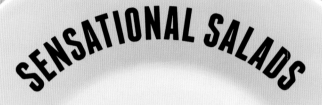

SENSATIONAL SALADS

All these nutritious, good-looking salads are light but filling. Just the kind of meal that is so perfect at lunch, which is often also a really great time to get the five-a-day box ticked. And they also work very well as side dishes to accompany meat or fish with an evening meal, or as colourful platters for sharing with a group of friends or family (just scale up the quantities to serve a crowd). A plate of one or more of our salads will give you all your five-a-day... and probably more. With so much variety in colour, texture and taste on offer, getting five-a-day is a doddle.

WARM INDIAN 'CHANA CHAAT' WITH POMEGRANATE | *serves 2*

This spicy salad is inspired by the Indian street food chana chaat. *Our spicy onion chutney enhances the delicate and subtle flavours of chickpea and aubergine, while the pomegranate and pumpkin seeds give a satisfying crunch.*

For the spicy onion chutney
a little sunflower oil
a few fresh curry leaves (leave them out
*   if you can't get fresh leaves)*
1 tsp cumin seeds
1 tsp mustard seeds
1 medium onion, finely sliced (160g)
1 heaped tbsp madras powder or paste
a little honey
1 tbsp cider vinegar

For the salad
1 small aubergine (160g)
160g sweet potato
1–2 tbsp sunflower oil
80g baby spinach
80g frozen peas
40g frozen edamame
1 tbsp pumpkin seeds
½ x 400g can of chickpeas, drained and
*   rinsed (net weight about 120g)*
large handful of chopped coriander
1 tbsp pomegranate seeds

5 OF YOUR 5-A-DAY

Preheat the oven to 200°C/fan 180°C/400°F/gas mark 6.

To make the chutney, heat a little oil in a pan and add the curry leaves, cumin and mustard seeds. When the seeds start to pop, add the onion, madras powder, a little honey, the vinegar and 50ml of water. Cover and leave to cook over a low heat for about one hour, or until you have a nice thick chutney, stirring and splashing in a bit of water now and again to stop the onion and spices catching. Leave to cool.

Meanwhile, cut the aubergine and the sweet potato into bite-sized pieces. Toss with the oil and roast for 30 minutes until soft. Remove from the oven and mix with the spinach so that it wilts a little. Pour hot water over the peas and edamame in a bowl to defrost them.

Tip the pumpkin seeds into a dry frying pan, set over a medium heat and stir for a minute or two, until they turn a shade darker and smell fragrant. Tip out on to a plate to stop the cooking.

In a large bowl, mix together the chickpeas, the drained peas and edamame, the roasted vegetables, spinach and coriander. Carefully stir through the spicy onion chutney.

Sprinkle with the pumpkin seeds and pomegranate seeds.

Serve with Cucumber and banana raita (see page 170) and your salad will climb to six portions.

Top Tip The chutney will keep in an airtight container in the fridge for five days and is the perfect accompaniment to all kinds of vegetables and salads.

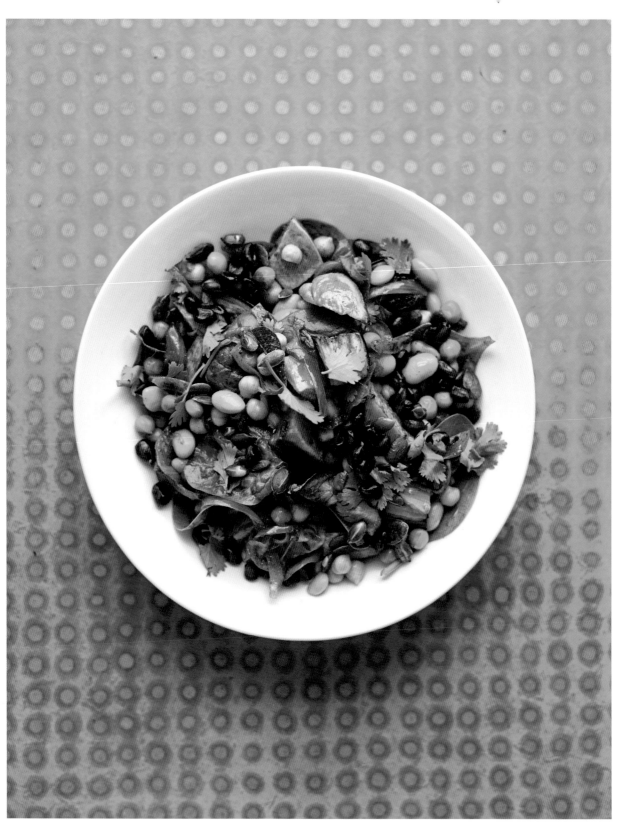

ROAST BEETROOT, SQUASH AND LENTIL SALAD WITH GOAT'S CHEESE | *serves 2*

A spectacular salad of vibrant colours and contrasting textures. Roasting the vegetables concentrates and sweetens their flavours, providing a perfect complement to the smooth and creamy goat's cheese.

1 large beetroot, peeled and cut into
    bite-sized pieces (160g)
1–2 tbsp olive oil, plus more to dress
¼ butternut squash, peeled and
    chopped into bite-sized pieces (160g)
1 large red onion, chopped into
    bite-sized pieces (160g)
60g green lentils or Puy lentils (about
    160g when cooked)
80g baby spinach
sea salt and freshly ground black pepper
80g frozen peas, defrosted
leaves from a small bunch of mint,
    finely chopped
small bunch of coriander,
    finely chopped
2 tbsp sunflower seeds (30g)
50g goat's cheese, or feta

**5 OF YOUR
5-A-DAY**

Preheat the oven to 200°C/fan 180°C/400°F/gas mark 6. Place the beetroot in a roasting tin, toss with the oil and roast for about 15 minutes. Add the butternut squash and red onion and continue roasting until all the vegetables are cooked but still firm, about another 40 minutes.

Meanwhile, rinse the lentils, then cook according to the packet instructions. They should still hold their shape, so be careful not to overcook them.

Put the spinach in a colander and tip the cooked lentils over the leaves so they wilt slightly. While warm, season with salt and pepper.

Mix the warm lentils with the peas and roasted vegetables, mint and coriander. Adjust the seasoning to taste.

Toast the sunflower seeds in a dry frying pan until golden. Sprinkle the seeds over the salad and crumble over the cheese and a little more olive oil, if you like.

Top Tip Spinach is a great way to up your five-a-day as it's easily added to salads, soups and curries. A whole heap of leaves will wilt down to a spoonful in seconds.

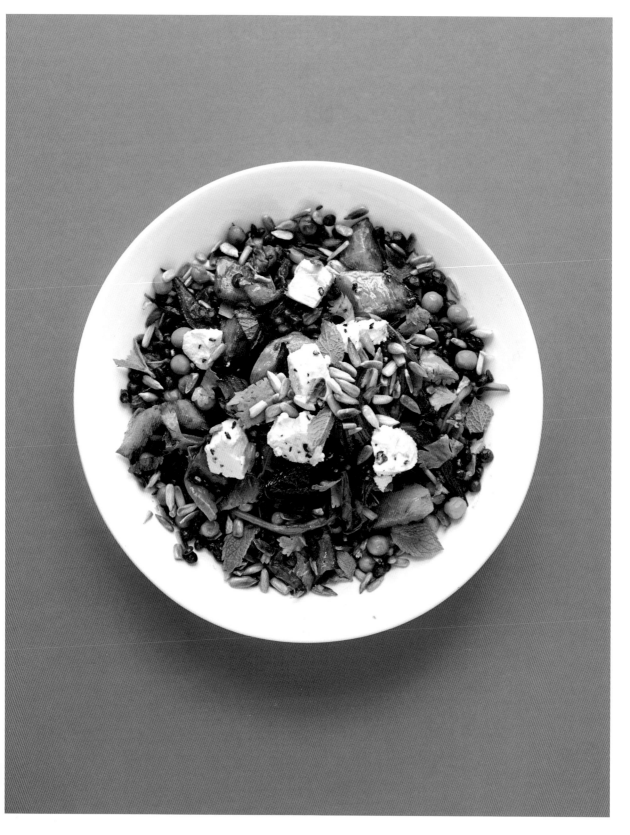

BULGAR AND CHARGRILLED VEGETABLE
SALAD WITH ONION JAM | *serves 2*

This hearty salad is inspired by the Greek flavours of feta, olives, thyme and honey. It combines the smoky taste of chargrilled vegetables with a scented sweet onion jam and is finished with mint. This is great served with grilled lamb chops.

For the onion jam
a little olive oil
1 medium onion, finely sliced (160g)
½ bulb of fennel, finely sliced (80g)
small bunch of thyme, tied with string
1 tbsp cider vinegar
1 tbsp runny honey
sea salt and freshly ground black pepper

For the salad
1 courgette, sliced lengthways (160g)
250g pack of asparagus spears, tough lower stems removed (should yield about 160g)
½ red pepper, sliced (80g)
70g bulgar wheat
1 heaped tbsp good-quality black olives, pitted and halved (20g)
60g sun-blushed tomatoes, or slow-roasted tomatoes (see right)
leaves from a small bunch of mint, finely chopped
50g feta cheese
2 tbsp sunflower seeds, toasted (see page 30)
a little extra virgin olive oil (optional)

5 OF YOUR 5-A-DAY

To make the jam, heat a little oil in a pan, add the onion, fennel, thyme, cider vinegar and honey with a pinch of salt. Cover and leave to cook over a low heat for about one hour, or until you have a thick, sweet jam, stirring and topping up with water now and again to stop the onion catching. Leave to cool. It will keep in the fridge in an airtight container for up to five days.

Meanwhile, heat a griddle until smoking and chargrill the courgette, asparagus and red pepper in turn. Cut the chargrilled vegetables into bite-sized pieces and set aside. Cook the bulgar wheat according to the packet instructions. Drain and season.

Mix the bulgar with the chargrilled vegetables, olives, tomatoes, onion jam and mint. Top with the feta and toasted sunflower seeds, adding a little extra virgin olive oil, if you like.

Slow-roasted tomatoes Preheat the oven to 130°C/fan 110°C/260°F/gas mark ¾. Halve a couple of punnets of cherry tomatoes, drizzle with olive oil and season with good-quality dried oregano, sea salt and freshly ground black pepper. Line a roasting tray with baking parchment and spread the tomatoes out, cut sides up. Roast in the oven for about two hours. Store in an airtight container in the fridge for up to three days. (160g of fresh tomatoes yields about 60g after slow-roasting.)

Top Tip When tomatoes are cheap towards the end of summer, slow-roasting them and using them in all kinds of dishes is a great way to up your five-a-day.

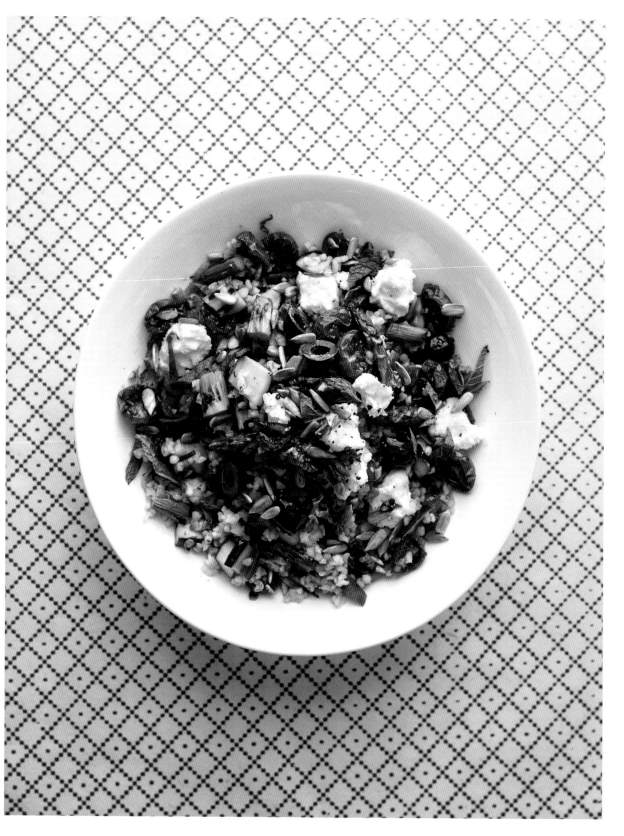

'TABBOULEH' WITH LENTILS, RED GRAPES AND FETA | *serves 2*

A Lebanese-inspired salad enhanced by lentils, peppers, grapes and sumac. This unique and eye-catching dish is certain to draw compliments from your guests. Our Sweet potato and courgette falafel are a perfect accompaniment (see page 138).

For the tabbouleh
*80g Puy lentils (about 160g
   when cooked)
sea salt and freshly ground black pepper
2 tbsp olive oil
½ small onion, finely chopped (40g)
½ medium carrot, finely chopped (40g)
2 large handfuls each of mint and
   parsley leaves, finely chopped
160g cherry tomatoes, halved
½ cucumber, deseeded and sliced on
   the diagonal (160g)
½ red pepper, cut into 1cm pieces (80g)
½ yellow pepper, cut into 1cm
   pieces (80g)
large handful of radishes, cut into thin
   rounds (80g)
small handful of red grapes, sliced
1 tsp sumac
50g feta cheese*

For the dressing
*75g natural yogurt
1 tsp runny honey
handful of finely chopped
   parsley and dill leaves
juice of ½ lemon*

Rinse the lentils, then cook according to the packet instructions. They should still hold their shape, so be careful not to overcook them. Drain and season with salt, pepper and a little olive oil.

Meanwhile, sauté the onion and carrot in the remaining olive oil until soft and sweet. While still warm, add a good handful of the mint and parsley and the cooked lentils. Set aside.

To make the dressing, mix all the ingredients in a bowl.

Combine the lentil mixture with the other vegetables and the grapes. Add the remaining herbs and season with sumac, salt and pepper. Mix well. Crumble over the feta and serve with the dressing on the side.

**5 OF YOUR
5-A-DAY**

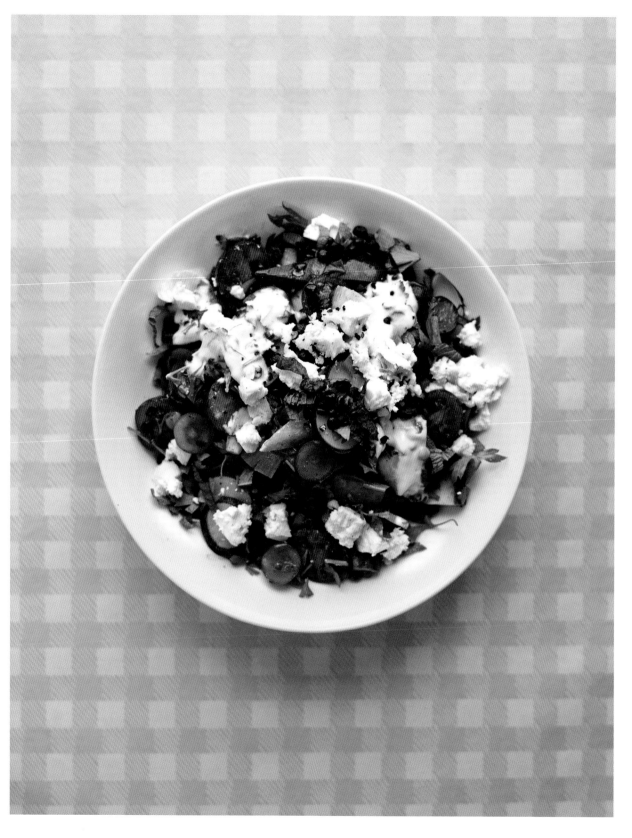

WARM ROASTED ROOTS WITH BUFFALO MOZZARELLA AND BALSAMIC | *serves 2*

Kohlrabi and mooli provide an interesting addition to the more common root vegetables used here. Their sweet, honeyed flavours are complemented by the tangy dressing and creamy cheese. A delicious dish which works well with roast chicken.

2 tbsp olive oil
4–5 sprigs of lemon thyme, or regular thyme
1 tbsp runny honey
2 garlic cloves, finely chopped
½ small swede (160g)
½ small kohlrabi (160g)
½ mooli or daikon (80g)
1 large carrot (160g)
sea salt and freshly ground black pepper
1 small parsnip (80g)
1 large beetroot (160g)
1 tbsp balsamic vinegar
2 large handfuls of rocket, baby spinach, or other salad leaves
125g buffalo mozzarella
1 tbsp chopped basil leaves

5 OF YOUR 5-A-DAY

Preheat the oven to 200°C/fan 180°C/400°F/gas mark 6.

Put half the oil in a mixing bowl, add the lemon thyme, honey and garlic. Mix well.

Peel and cut the swede, kohlrabi and mooli into 2–3cm wedges. Cut the carrot on the diagonal into 5mm slices. Add to the bowl and coat with the marinade.

Line two baking trays with foil. Leaving as much of the marinade in the bowl as possible, spread the marinated roots evenly across one of the trays and sprinkle with salt. Roast for one hour, turning everything about halfway through.

In the meantime, peel and cut the parsnip and beetroot into 2–3cm wedges. Ensuring you keep them separate (so that the beetroot does not colour the parsnip), firstly coat the parsnip in some of the remaining marinade and place on the second baking tray. Repeat with the beetroot and the remaining marinade. Roast for 40 minutes, turning halfway through.

Mix the remaining oil and the balsamic to make a dressing.

Put the salad leaves in a serving dish. Remove the lemon thyme stalks from the vegetables and place everything (except the beetroot) on top of the leaves. Pour over the dressing, making sure all the vegetables are well coated. Season with salt and pepper. Carefully place the beetroot over the other vegetables. Break the mozzarella over the warm salad and finish with the basil leaves.

Note If you can't find kohlrabi, simply double the quantity of parsnip and mooli, or include some turnip instead.

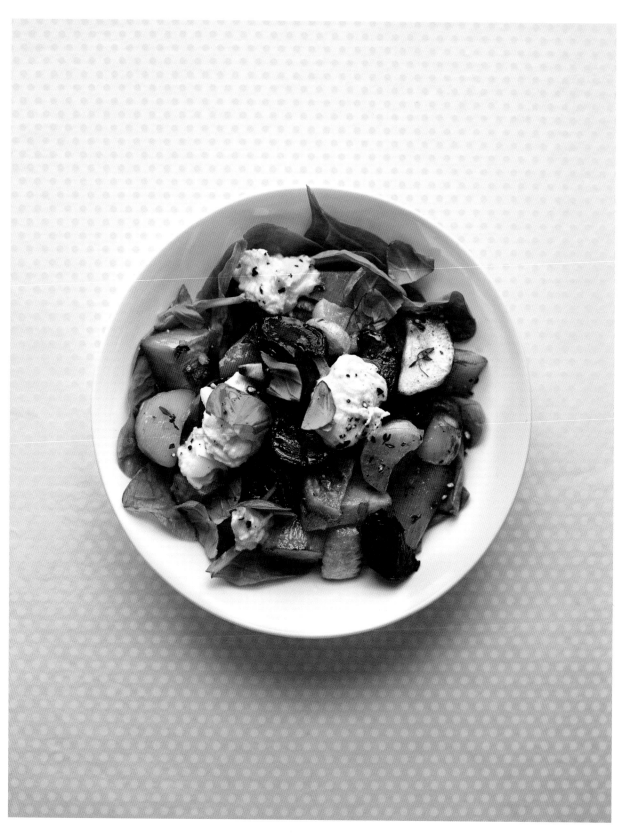

THAI GREEN PAPAYA SALAD | *serves 2*

This is a perfect dinner party salad, as it benefits from being left to steep for up to two hours. (Obviously just scale up the proportions to serve more people.) The zingy lime, ginger and chilli dressing makes this so moreish that it rarely makes it to the table without half being devoured! Delicious with grilled prawns or chicken satay.

For the salad
1 small green papaya (80g)
½ cucumber, deseeded (160g)
1 large carrot (160g)
1 red pepper (160g)
handful of mange tout (80g)
10cm piece of mooli or daikon (80g)
handful of beansprouts (80g)
large handful of chopped coriander
finely grated zest and juice of 1 lime
sprinkling of peanuts or sesame
    seeds (optional)

For the dressing
1 tsp sunflower oil
2 tsp sesame oil
2 tbsp light soy sauce
2 tsp rice vinegar
1 tbsp kecap manis, or 1 tbsp palm sugar
1 tsp finely chopped root ginger
1 small red chilli,
    finely chopped

5 OF YOUR
5-A-DAY

Peel the papaya and cut in half lengthways. Remove the black seeds and slice the flesh thinly using a mandolin or sharp knife, before cutting it into matchsticks. (Or use a julienner.)

Cut the cucumber into matchsticks, together with the carrot, pepper and mange tout. Finely shred the mooli and mix everything in a bowl with the beansprouts and coriander.

For the dressing, mix together all the ingredients, pour over the salad and toss gently. Leave to steep in the fridge for at least 30 minutes. Meanwhile, roast the peanuts or sesame seeds (if using) in a dry frying pan set over a medium heat until coloured. Tip into a bowl to stop the cooking.

Just before serving, toss in the lime zest and juice and top with the peanuts or sesame seeds.

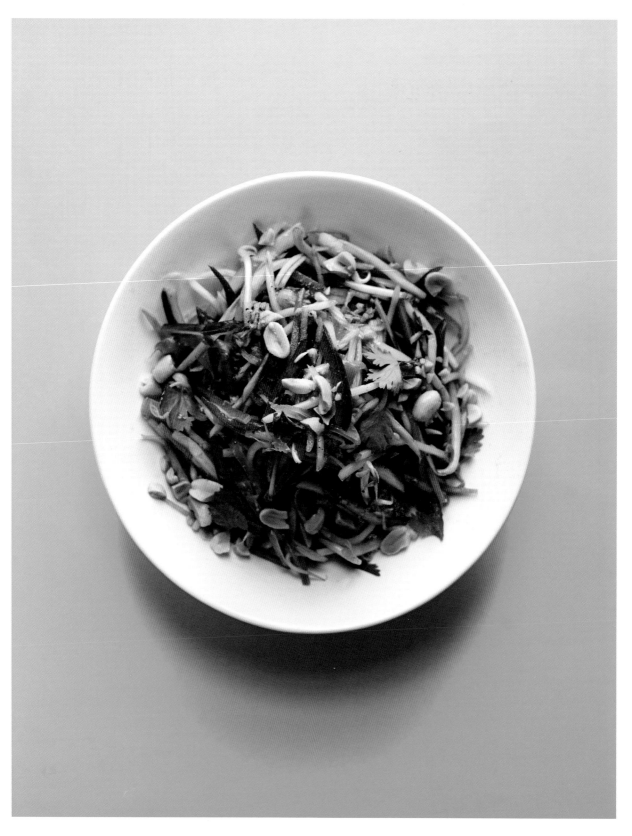

FRUITY QUINOA SALAD | *serves 2*

A dish full of vibrant colour, this combines the contrasting textures of mango and dried fruit with crunchy raw vegetables, so it's hard to resist. The addition of zingy lemon and mint make it really refreshing, too. Great with roast chicken.

80g mixed quinoa (or red quinoa and
  bulgar wheat)
1 red pepper, finely chopped (160g)
½ cucumber, deseeded and finely
  chopped (160g)
1 small carrot, finely chopped (80g)
½ mango, cut into cubes (80g)
seeds from ½ pomegranate (80g)
4 dried apricots, coarsely chopped (40g)
1 heaped tbsp dried cranberries,
  chopped
2 large handfuls of mint leaves,
  finely chopped
sea salt and freshly ground black pepper
80g mixed leaves, or baby spinach
1–2 tbsp olive oil
juice of 1 lemon
1 large avocado (160g)

5 OF YOUR 5-A-DAY

Wash the quinoa, or the quinoa and bulgar wheat, and cook according to the packet instructions. Drain and set aside.

Mix all the prepared vegetables and fruit, except the avocado, with the cooked quinoa, then stir through the mint. Season with salt and pepper and mix with the leaves. Add the oil and half the lemon juice.

Just before serving, cut half the avocado into chunks and mix into the salad. Slice the other half and toss in the remaining lemon juice to stop the slices from discolouring. Lay them over the salad.

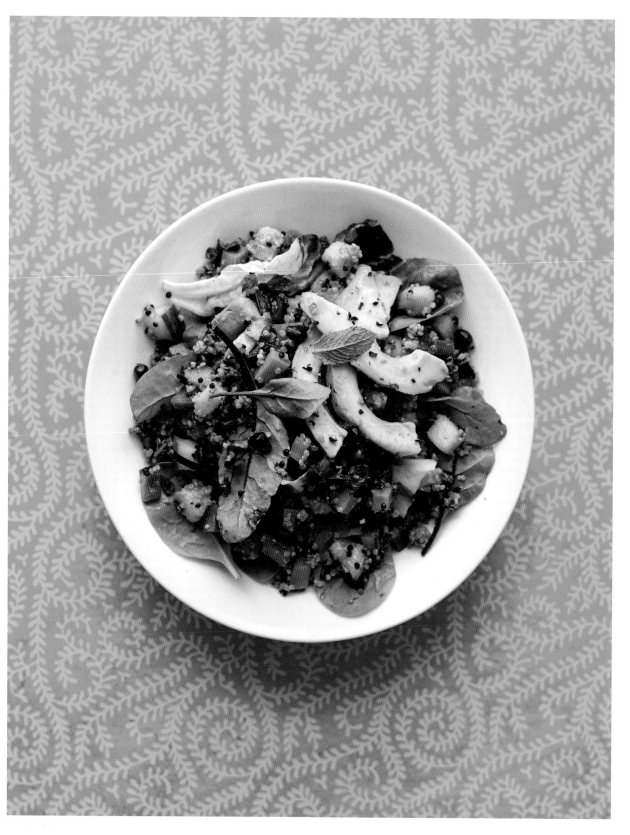

TANGY FENNEL AND ARTICHOKE SALAD
WITH OLIVES AND CAPER BERRIES | serves 2

A great alternative to a Greek salad. The large caper berries provide a salty and tangy contrast to the sweetness of the roasted vegetables. This is good alongside white fish.

½ fennel bulb, cut into bite-sized
  pieces (80g)
1 large red onion, cut into bite-sized
  pieces (160g)
160g chestnut mushrooms, cut into
  bite-sized pieces
1 courgette, cut into bite-sized
  pieces (160g)
½ red pepper, cut into bite-sized
  pieces (80g)
2 tbsp olive oil
a few thyme leaves
sea salt and freshly ground black pepper
80g wild rice
handful of cherry tomatoes,
  halved (80g)
4 marinated artichoke hearts, cut into
  bite-sized pieces
80g black and green olives, halved
12 large caper berries
finely grated zest and juice of
  1 unwaxed lemon
handful of basil leaves
4 tbsp roughly chopped
  parsley leaves

5 OF YOUR
5-A-DAY

Preheat the oven to 200°C/fan 180°C/400°F/gas mark 6.

Place the fennel, onion, mushrooms, courgette and red pepper in a roasting tray, drizzle with the oil, sprinkle on the thyme, salt and pepper and roast for about 45 minutes until all the vegetables are cooked. Stir halfway through.

Meanwhile, cook the rice according to packet instructions. Drain and set aside.

When the vegetables are cooked, mix in the tomatoes, artichokes, olives, caper berries and lemon zest. Now mix these with the rice and stir in the lemon juice and herbs.

Serve warm or cold.

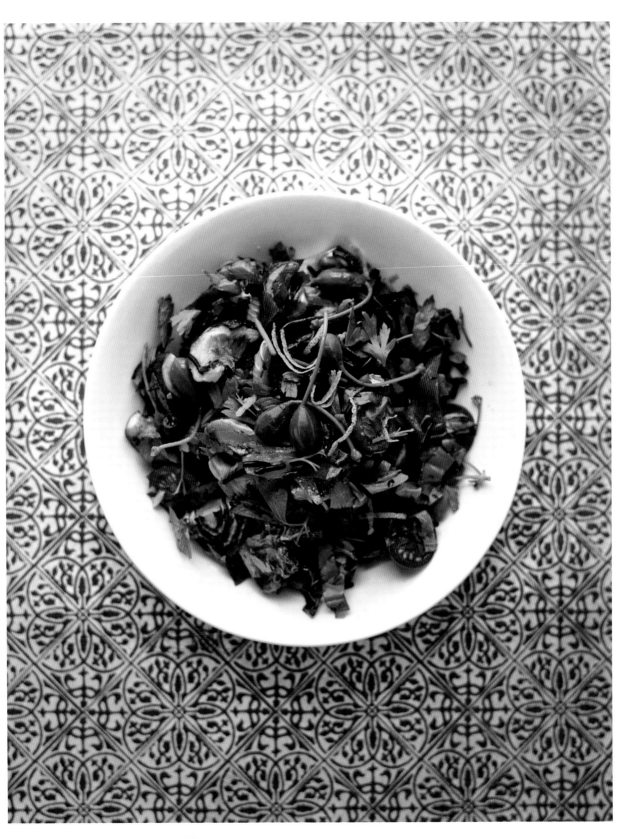

SPICY COUSCOUS BOWL | *serves 2*

The inclusion of harissa and cumin give this aubergine, courgette and pepper salad a spicy North African influence. The coriander and mint enhance the flavour of the couscous, while providing a fine complement to the spices in this dish.

1 small aubergine (160g)
1 yellow pepper (160g)
80g mushrooms
1 courgette (160g)
1 medium onion (160g)
2 tbsp extra virgin olive oil
2 tbsp harissa paste
3 tsp cumin seeds
sea salt and freshly ground black pepper
100g couscous
½ tsp vegetable bouillon powder
4 tbsp finely chopped coriander
4 tbsp finely chopped parsley leaves
large handful of cherry tomatoes, halved (80g)
finely grated zest and juice of
   1 unwaxed lemon

5 OF YOUR 5-A-DAY

Preheat the oven to 200°C/fan 180°C/400°F/gas mark 6.

Cut all the vegetables, except the cherry tomatoes, into bite-sized pieces and place in a roasting tray with the oil, harissa, cumin seeds, salt and pepper. Roast for about 40 minutes until cooked, turning halfway through.

Meanwhile, make the couscous by placing in a bowl, mixing in the bouillon powder and covering with 150ml of boiling water. Cover tightly with cling film and leave for five minutes. Once cooked, fluff the couscous with a fork.

Take the vegetables out of the oven and, while still warm, add the herbs and tomatoes.

Mix the vegetables with the couscous – or simply serve the vegetables on top of a bed of couscous – and season with salt and pepper. Add the lemon zest and juice and mix together to serve.

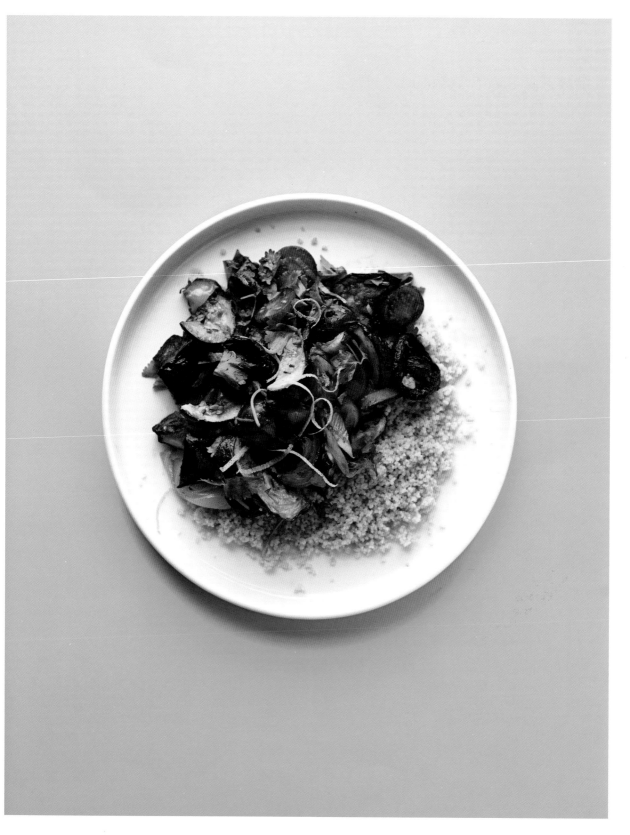

WARM DOUBLE PEAR SALAD WITH BLUE CHEESE AND WALNUTS | *serves 2*

This classic combination of sweet pear, tangy blue cheese and crunchy walnuts has been enhanced with rocket and creamy avocado to make it a really luxurious five-a-day dish. If you like a stronger cheese, you could use Roquefort or Stilton.

For the dressing
1 tbsp sunflower oil
½ large red onion, finely chopped (80g)
2 small celery sticks, finely
    chopped (80g)
2 tbsp wholegrain mustard
juice of ½ lemon

For the salad
250g pack of asparagus spears, tough
    lower stems removed (should yield
    about 160g)
½ large tart apple, such as Granny
    Smith (80g)
1 large pear (160g)
1 tsp sunflower oil
1 tbsp salted butter
½ tsp finely chopped rosemary
40g rocket
40g watercress
50g mild blue cheese, such as
    Gorgonzola
1 large avocado (160g)
40g walnuts, chopped

**5 OF YOUR
5-A-DAY**

For the dressing, heat the oil in a pan and fry the onion and celery for seven to 10 minutes until soft. Add the mustard and lemon juice and set aside.

Meanwhile, cook the asparagus in gently simmering water for two to three minutes. Drain and pat dry.

Core the apple and pear and cut into 5mm slices. Heat the 1 tsp of oil in a large frying pan, add the slices and cook for two minutes, turning carefully halfway through.

Preheat the grill to a medium setting. In a separate ovenproof frying pan, heat the butter until golden. Add the rosemary and asparagus. Sauté for a couple of minutes before adding half the rocket and half the watercress. Mix briefly and crumble the cheese over the top. Place under the grill for about three minutes, until the cheese is melted and the asparagus glazed.

Now arrange the salad by placing the remaining rocket and watercress in a bowl. Slice the avocado and place on top, then add the lukewarm apple and pear slices. Top with the warm asparagus and cheese mixture, spoon over the dressing and finish with the chopped walnuts. Serve warm.

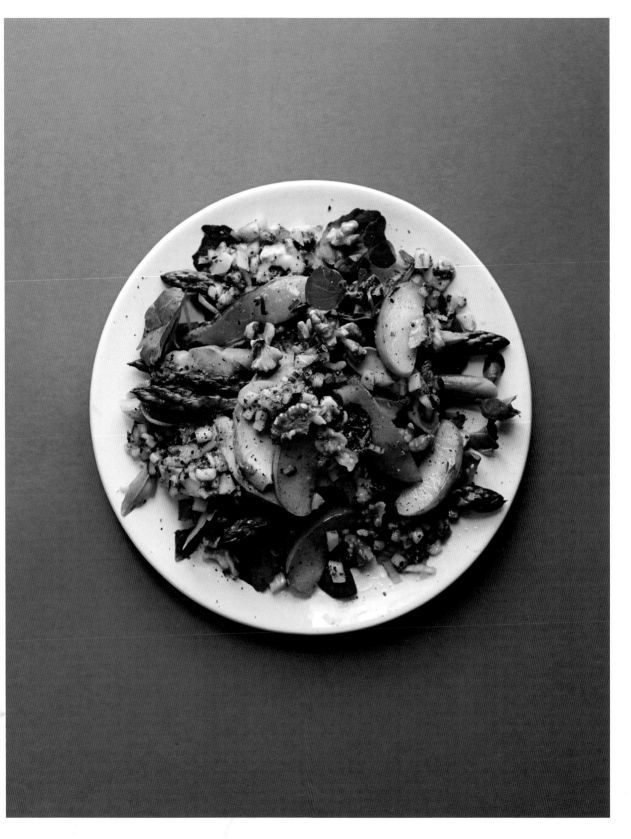

GADO GADO | *serves 2*

The name of this salad means 'mix mix' and it can be made with raw or cooked vegetables. In keeping with tradition, we suggest serving the dish with boiled eggs and crispy shallots. Our spicy Indonesian peanut sauce will keep in the fridge for a few days and complements many different vegetables.

For the spicy peanut sauce
2 tbsp crunchy peanut butter
½ tsp shrimp paste (optional)
1 tsp kecap manis
1 tsp white wine vinegar
1½ tsp tamarind paste
1½ tsp brown sugar
¼ tsp salt
1 tsp groundnut oil
1–2 red chillies, finely chopped
   (with seeds if you like it hot)
1 garlic clove, finely chopped
100ml coconut milk

For the salad
1 tbsp groundnut oil
2 banana shallots, finely sliced (80g)
2 eggs
1 large carrot, cut in fine batons (160g)
½ cucumber, deseeded and sliced on
   the diagonal (160g)
¼ head of Chinese leaf, shredded (80g)
handful of beansprouts (80g)
1 red pepper, finely sliced (160g)
2 small celery sticks, sliced (80g)
2 tbsp salted peanuts,
   roughly chopped

Place the peanut butter in a food processor. Wrap the shrimp paste in foil and toast for a couple of minutes in a dry frying pan, turning halfway through. Unwrap and add the shrimp paste to the food processor with the kecap manis, vinegar, tamarind, sugar, salt and 1 tbsp of hot water.

Add the oil, chillies and garlic to another pan and heat gently for a couple of minutes until cooked, but not coloured. Add to the food processor. Process everything until well blended, scraping the mixture from the sides if necessary. Add the coconut milk and blend for a final minute. Pour the sauce into a serving bowl.

For the salad, heat the oil in a pan and add the shallots. Cook for 10–12 minutes until brown and crisp.

Meanwhile heat some water in a pan and, once it boils, carefully add the eggs and simmer gently for about five minutes. Drain and carefully peel them.

Arrange the salad vegetables on a plate, place the halved eggs on top and scatter over the crispy shallots and salted peanuts. Serve with the spicy peanut sauce.

**5 OF YOUR
5-A-DAY**

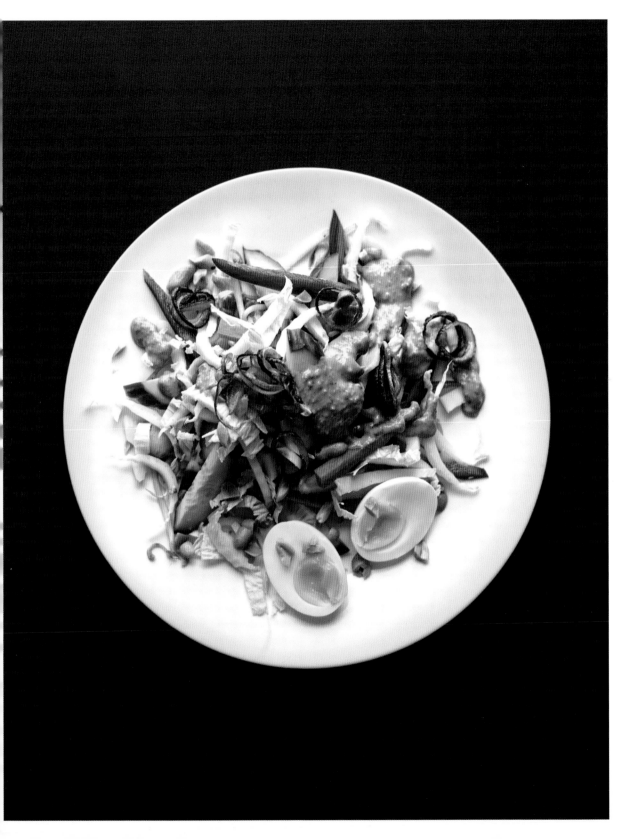

MEAL-IN-A-BOWL SOUPS

Eating a bowl of nourishing soup is one of the easiest ways to get all your five-a-day into a single meal. Whether you fancy something creamy and smooth, chunky and spicy, steaming hot or refreshingly chilled, there's a recipe in this chapter to suit every mood or occasion. Making soup is also a great way to use up leftover vegetables. Rather than leaving them languishing at the bottom of the fridge at the end of the week, or letting them go to waste, cook and blend them into one of these tasty and substantial dishes.

MALAYSIAN LAKSA WITH COURGETTE 'NOODLES' | *serves 2*

This light, colourful and mildly spiced soup introduces the idea of courgette 'noodles'. To create a more substantial dish, simply add your preferred type of regular noodles. You could also put in some prawns or strips of chicken, if you like.

160g sweet potato, cut into 1cm cubes
2 tbsp sunflower oil
1 medium onion, finely chopped (160g)
2 kaffir lime leaves, very finely chopped
1 lemon grass stalk, bruised
2 tbsp Madras curry paste
1 tsp Thai red curry paste
80g chestnut mushrooms, cut into
　bite-sized pieces
handful of broccoli florets, stem peeled
　and cut into bite-sized pieces (80g)
400ml can of coconut milk
300ml vegetable or chicken stock
handful of sugar snap peas, cut into
　bite-sized pieces (80g)
1 small head of pak choi, chopped (80g)
1 courgette, made into noodles with a
　'spiraliser' or julienner (160g)
1 tsp sesame oil
large handful of chopped coriander
sea salt and freshly ground black pepper

To serve
small handful of beansprouts
½ red chilli, finely chopped
lime wedges

Preheat the oven to 180°C/fan 160°C/350°F/gas mark 4. Spread the sweet potato on a baking sheet, toss in 1 tbsp of the oil and roast for 20 minutes or until just cooked (this helps to improve its flavour).

Fry the onion, kaffir lime leaves and lemon grass with the two curry pastes in the remaining 1 tbsp of oil for a few minutes, adding a little water to ensure the pastes don't burn. When the onion is soft, add the mushrooms and broccoli stems and fry for a few more minutes.

Add the coconut milk and stock and simmer for about 20 minutes. Once the flavours have infused, add the broccoli florets, sugar snap peas and pak choi and continue to cook until just tender but still retaining a firm bite. Lastly, add the sweet potato and courgette noodles and cook for a final two minutes before adding the sesame oil and coriander.

Season to taste and serve in bowls topped with crunchy beansprouts, red chilli and lime wedges.

Top Tip It's worth investing in a hand-held julienner or spiraliser as it will come in handy for all types of dishes. It will transform the appearance of your vegetables and give them a real 'wow' factor.

5 OF YOUR 5-A-DAY

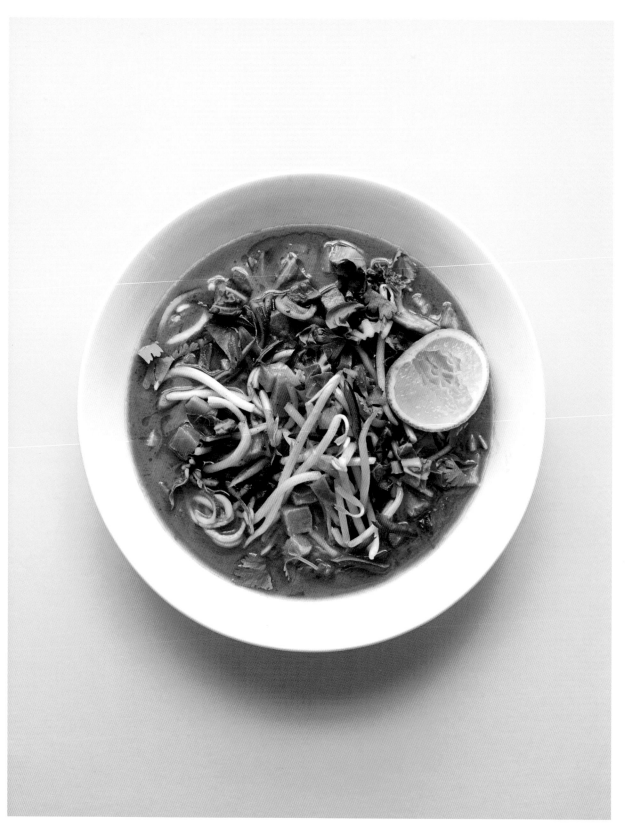

CURRIED RED LENTIL, SPINACH AND COCONUT BROTH | *serves 2*

Our hearty and substantial curry soup recipe is a meal in itself; it's delightfully colourful and has warm, subtle spicing. Great on its own or served with naan bread.

1 small carrot, roughly chopped (80g)
2 small celery sticks, roughly chopped (80g)
1 garlic clove
1 tbsp sunflower oil
1 tsp cumin seeds
1 tsp mustard seeds
1 medium onion, finely chopped (160g)
½ red pepper, chopped (80g)
small bunch of coriander, stalks finely chopped and leaves roughly chopped
sea salt and freshly ground black pepper
1 tsp ground cumin
1 tsp ground coriander
1 tsp ground ginger
½ tsp ground turmeric
½ tsp chilli powder
90g red lentils (yields about 160g when cooked)
100ml coconut milk
500ml vegetable stock
2 large handfuls of cherry tomatoes (160g)
80g baby spinach

5 OF YOUR 5-A-DAY

Finely blitz the carrot, celery and garlic in a food processor.

Heat the oil in a heavy-based saucepan, add the cumin and mustard seeds and cook for about 30 seconds or until the mustard seeds start to pop. Add the onion, red pepper and coriander stalks to the pan with a little salt and cook for about eight minutes until soft.

Add the dry spices, the carrot and celery mixture and continue cooking for a further five minutes, adding a little water if the mixture threatens to catch.

Rinse the lentils thoroughly and add to the pan with the coconut milk and stock. Cook for 20 minutes or until the lentils are soft, topping up with hot water if necessary to reach your preferred consistency.

Add the cherry tomatoes and cook for about two minutes until just softened, take off the heat and stir in the spinach and coriander leaves, which will wilt in the residual warmth. Season with salt and pepper.

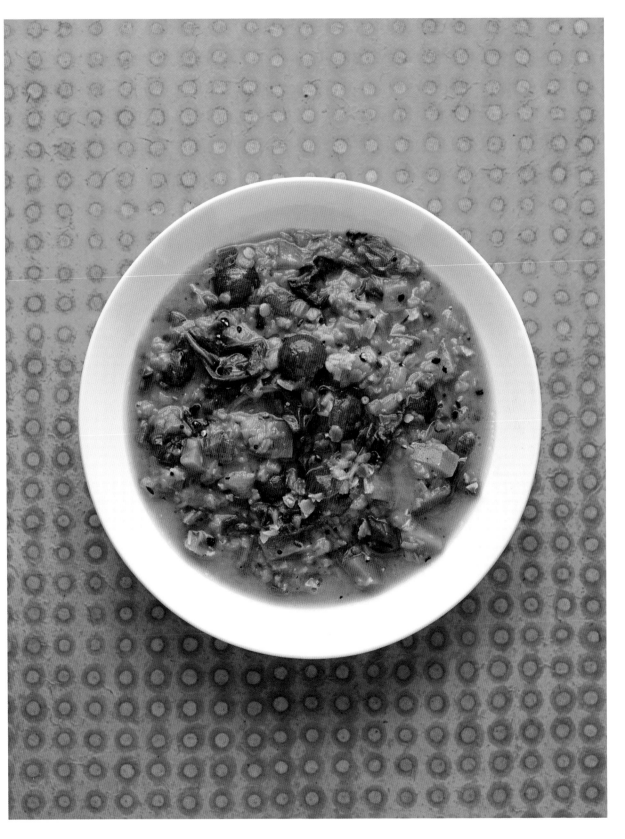

ROAST GAZPACHO | *serves 2*

This is a twist on the Andalusian classic, using roasted vegetables to enhance the flavour. It's a delicious and refreshing cold soup, best served on a hot summer's day with crusty French bread.

½ courgette (80g)
1 red pepper (160g)
1 small onion (80g)
2 small celery sticks (80g)
½ cucumber, deseeded (160g)
2–3 large tomatoes (200g)
1 small leek, trimmed (80g)
1 garlic clove, left whole, skin on
2 tbsp olive oil, plus more to serve
sea salt and freshly ground black pepper
500ml tomato juice
large handful of basil leaves
large handful of parsley leaves
good squeeze of lemon juice
a few shakes of Tabasco
2 tsp Worcestershire sauce

5 OF YOUR 5-A-DAY

Preheat the oven to 200°C/fan 180°C/400°F/gas mark 6. Cut all the vegetables into bite-sized pieces and spread evenly in a deep baking tray, tossing with the whole garlic clove and olive oil. Season with salt and pepper and roast in the oven for about 30 minutes.

When the vegetables are cooked, remove the skin from the garlic clove and place everything in a blender with the tomato juice, basil and parsley (reserve a few small basil leaves). You may need to do this in two batches. Season with more salt if required, black pepper, lemon juice, and the Tabasco and Worcestershire sauces. Blitz, then repeat to blitz the remaining soup, if necessary.

Chill in the fridge for at least 30 minutes or until ready to serve. The soup will be quite thick, but pour it into two serving bowls and add an ice cube to each; this will thin it a little.

Before serving, drizzle with a little more olive oil and top with the reserved basil leaves.

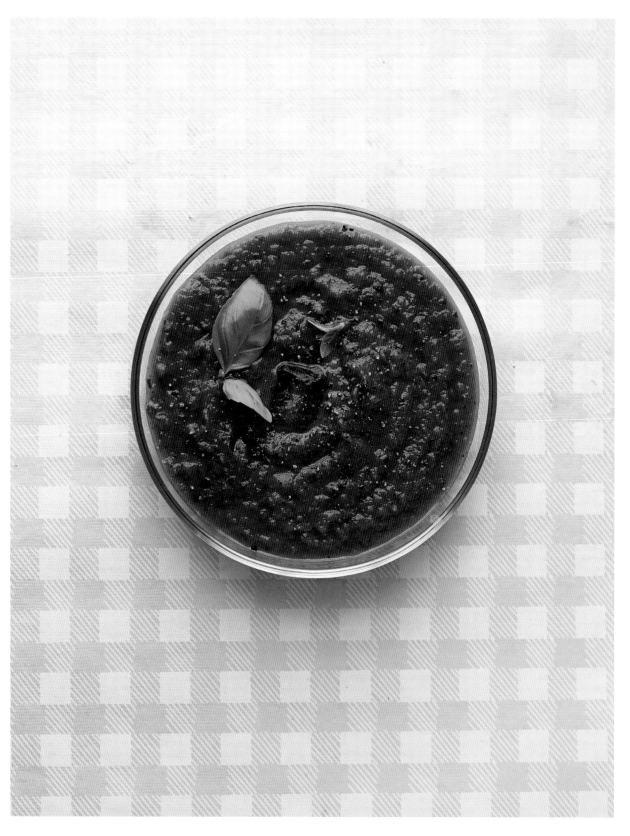

FRAGRANT CAULIFLOWER SOUP WITH COCONUT AND LEMON GRASS | *serves 2*

White in colour, this rich and luxurious soup indulges the senses despite its calm appearance. The combination of cauliflower and coconut creates a delicious and unique flavour. Make it, sup it and see for yourself!

1 medium onion (160g)
2 small leeks, trimmed, white parts only
   (160g)
4 small celery sticks (160g)
½ cauliflower (160g)
2 small turnips, peeled (160g)
1 tbsp sunflower oil
2 lemon grass stalks, tough outer leaves
   removed, finely chopped
400ml can of coconut milk
300ml vegetable stock
sea salt and freshly ground white pepper
good squeeze of lemon juice
a little olive oil, to serve

5 OF YOUR
5-A-DAY

Cut all the vegetables into small even-sized pieces.

Heat the sunflower oil in a large heavy-based saucepan and fry the onion, leeks and celery over a low heat for about 10 minutes, stirring constantly to ensure the vegetables do not brown. Add the cauliflower (reserving a few small florets), turnips and lemon grass and cook for a further five minutes, again ensuring nothing colours.

Add the coconut milk and stock and cook, uncovered, for about 12 minutes, until all the vegetables are soft.

Place the vegetables in a blender with the cooking liquid (you'll need to do this in two batches) and blend for a few minutes to get a smooth soup. Return to the pan and heat gently. Season with salt and white pepper and a good squeeze of lemon juice.

To serve, toast the reserved cauliflower florets in a dry frying pan and place on top of the soup with a drizzle of olive oil.

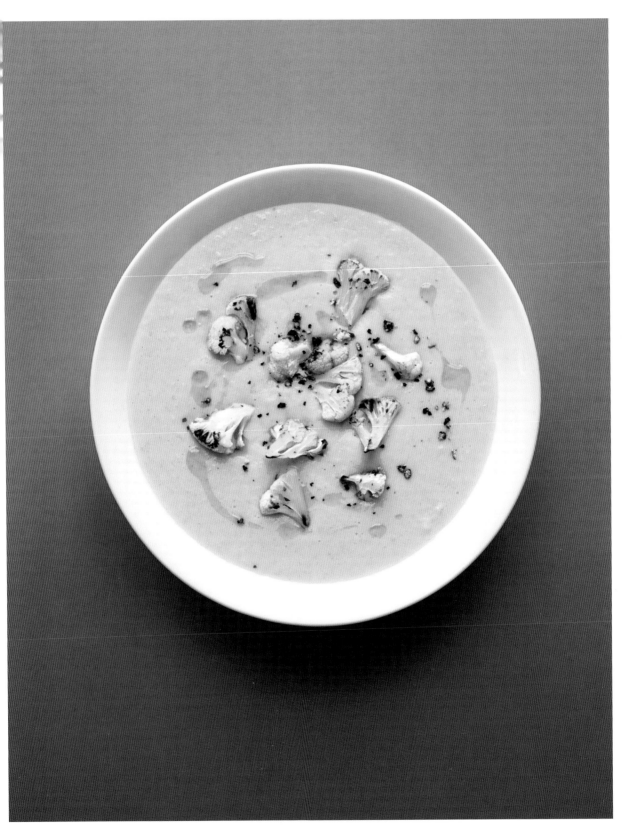

MINTED GREEN GARDEN SOUP | *serves 2*

A vibrant green soup full of vitality and bursting with summer flavours. The addition of mint provides a subtle freshness. It's very easy to make and incredibly healthy, too!

1 tbsp sunflower oil
1 medium onion, finely chopped (160g)
1 courgette, roughly chopped (160g)
½ large cucumber, deseeded and
   roughly chopped (160g)
about 400ml vegetable stock
160g frozen petits pois
160g baby spinach
handful of mint leaves, chopped
sea salt and freshly ground black pepper
1 tbsp lemon juice
½ tsp caster sugar (optional)

**5 OF YOUR
5-A-DAY**

Heat the oil in a heavy-based saucepan and fry the onion for about eight minutes until translucent. Add the courgette and cucumber, followed by the stock. Cover and simmer for a further 10 minutes until the courgette is cooked.

Add the peas and cook for two minutes before stirring in the spinach and mint for 30 seconds, just long enough for the leaves to wilt but also allow the peas to retain their bright green colour.

Place in a blender (you'll need to do this in two batches) and blend until smooth. Season with salt, pepper, lemon juice and sugar (you'll only need this if your petits pois weren't sweet).

Return to the pan and heat gently to serve.

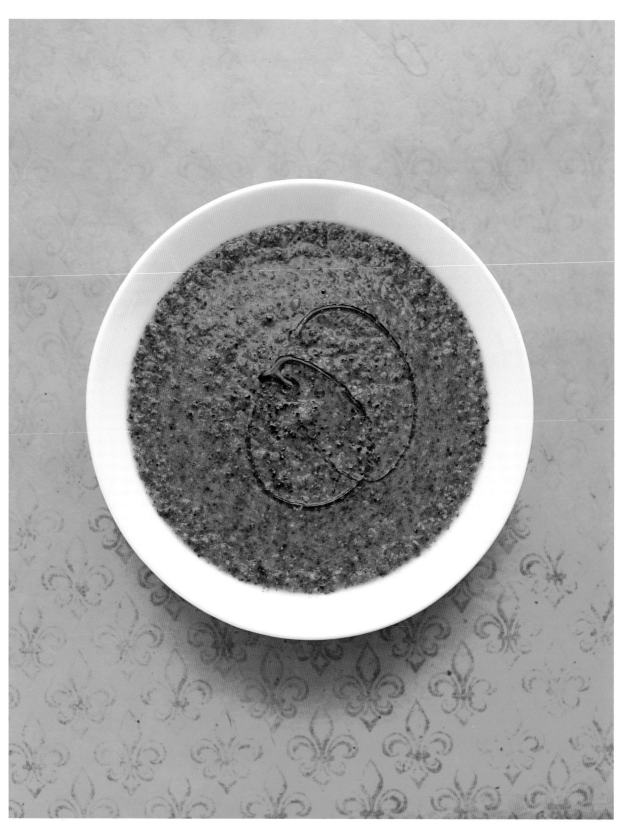

BROCCOLI, FENNEL AND STILTON SOUP | *serves 2*

Smooth, thick and creamy, this sumptuous soup is a twist on a British favourite. The fennel adds a very subtle flavour which we think enhances this classic dish but, if it's not to your taste, just add more broccoli.

1 medium onion (160g)
2 small celery sticks (80g)
1 large leek, trimmed (160g)
1 small carrot (80g)
1 fennel bulb (160g)
½ head of broccoli, florets removed
   from stems (160g)
1 tbsp sunflower oil
about 500ml vegetable stock, plus more
   if needed
1 bouquet garni (optional)
30g Stilton cheese
sea salt and freshly ground black pepper
handful of chives, chopped

5 OF YOUR 5-A-DAY

Cut all the vegetables into small even-sized pieces, including the broccoli stem (peel off the tough outer layer first).

Heat the oil in a heavy-based saucepan and sweat all the vegetables (except the broccoli florets), without colouring, for about 10 minutes.

Add the broccoli florets and just enough vegetable stock to cover the vegetables. Add the bouquet garni, if using, cover with a lid and simmer gently for about 15 minutes, or until the vegetables are cooked.

Place in a blender and blend until really smooth (you'll need to do this in two batches). Return to the pan, stir in half the Stilton and adjust the consistency by adding a little more stock if required. Heat slowly, seasoning to taste.

Serve in bowls with the remaining Stilton crumbled on top, sprinkled with the chives and a grind more black pepper, if you like.

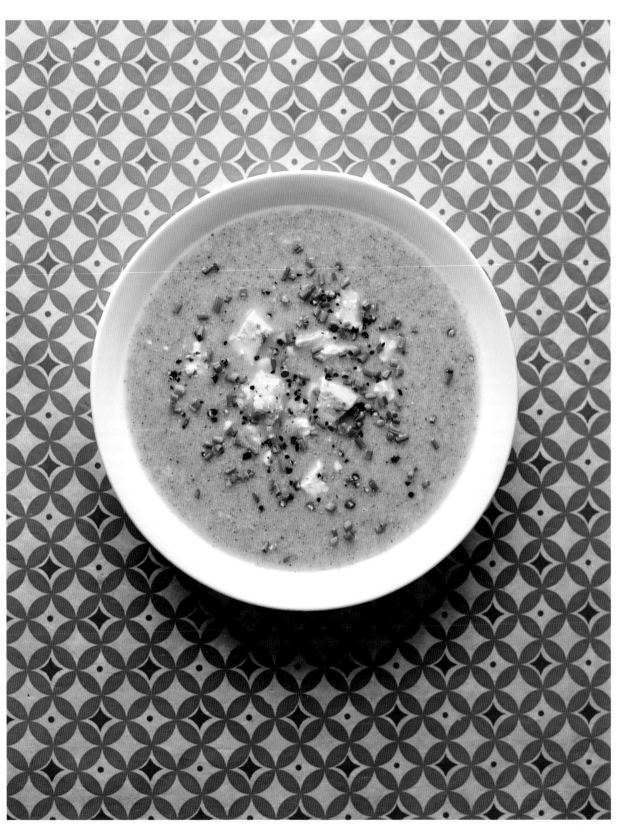

CARROT AND SWEET POTATO SOUP
WITH CHILLI AND CUMIN | *serves 2*

A wholesome, mildly spiced and warming soup. This is a versatile recipe to which additional or leftover vegetables can easily be added. We often add chilli to create a spicier soup but, if you don't like the heat, just leave it out.

1 medium onion (160g)
1 large leek, trimmed (160g)
1 large carrot (160g)
160g sweet potato
4 small celery sticks (160g)
1 tbsp sunflower oil
1 bay leaf
1 tbsp cumin seeds
½ red chilli, finely chopped (optional)
about 500ml vegetable stock, plus
    more if needed
sea salt and freshly ground black pepper
large handful of chopped coriander
a little olive oil (optional)
1 tsp single cream (optional)

**5 OF YOUR
5-A-DAY**

Cut all the vegetables into small even-sized pieces.

Heat the oil in a heavy-based saucepan and fry the bay leaf and cumin seeds until the seeds turn a shade darker and smell aromatic. Add the onion, chilli, if using, and leek and fry for about five minutes, stirring now and again. Add the carrot, sweet potato and celery and enough vegetable stock to cover. Season with salt and pepper, cover and cook for about 20 minutes until all the vegetables are tender.

Remove the bay leaf and transfer the vegetables to a blender with the coriander, reserving a few leaves (you'll need to blend the soup in two batches). Blend until smooth, adding a little more stock if necessary. Season to taste.

Serve in bowls with a drizzle of olive oil and a swirl of cream, if using, and topped with the reserved coriander leaves and a grind of black pepper, if you like.

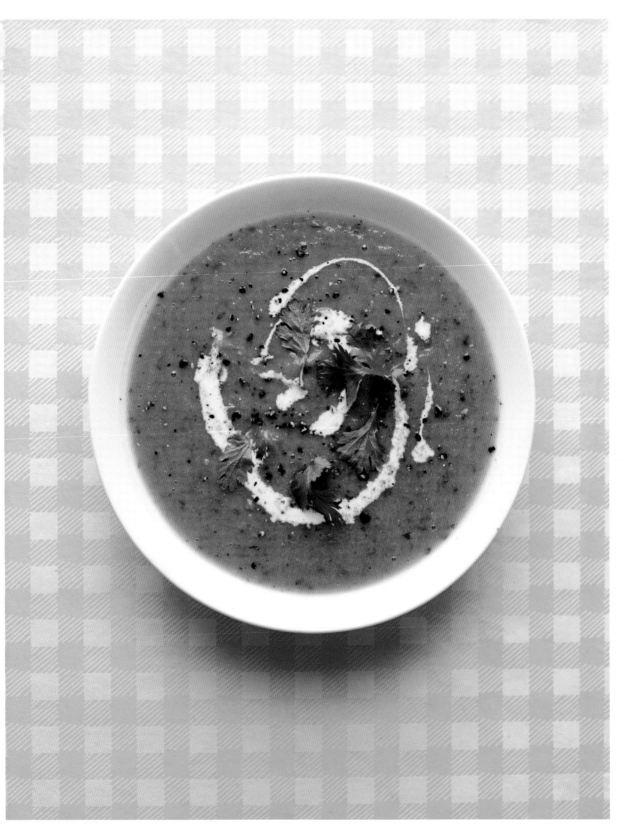

CORN CHOWDER WITH GREEN PEPPERS | *serves 2*

Traditionally a creamy potato-based soup, our recipe uses green pepper to complement the corn and give a really nutritious, colourful soup. Adding the crunchy green pepper at the end gives the soup a great texture.

1 medium onion (160g)
2 small celery sticks (80g)
1 small carrot (80g)
1 large leek, trimmed (160g)
1 green pepper (160g)
1 tbsp sunflower oil
1 bay leaf
3 sage leaves, roughly chopped
sea salt and freshly ground
  black pepper
160g canned or frozen sweetcorn
  (drained or defrosted)
250ml semi-skimmed milk
150ml vegetable stock
a touch of double cream or
  crème fraîche (optional)

5 OF YOUR 5-A-DAY

Finely chop the onion, celery, carrot, leek and green pepper. Set the green pepper aside.

Heat the oil in a saucepan, add the onion, celery, carrot and leek, bay leaf and sage leaves. Sweat with a pinch of salt for about 10 minutes. Add half the sweetcorn. Pour over the milk and stock, cover and cook gently for five to eight minutes.

Remove the bay leaf and blend for a couple of minutes using a hand-held blender. Add the green pepper, remaining sweetcorn and cream, if using. Season to taste and heat through gently to serve.

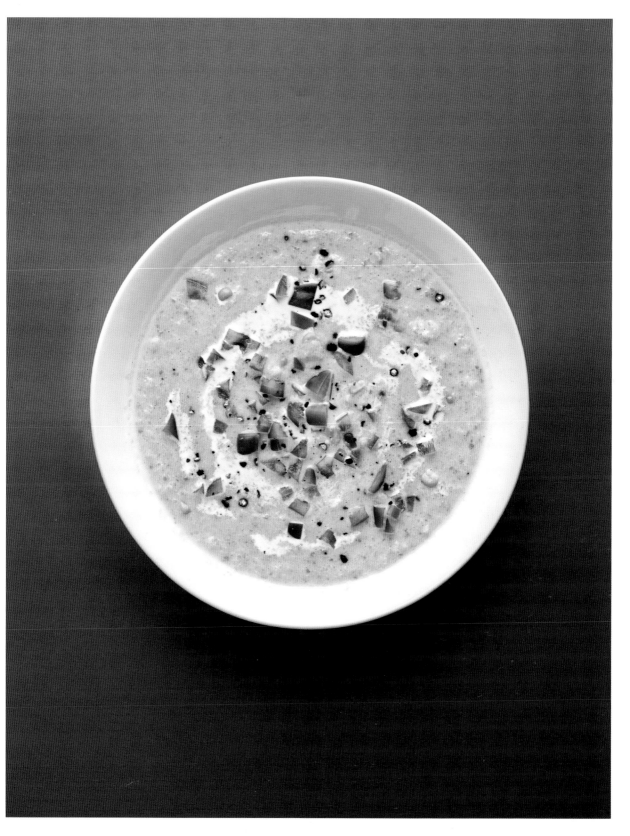

SPICY THAI COCONUT SOUP | serves 2

Our light and spicy soup uses traditional Thai ingredients: lemon grass, chilli, coconut and lime. It is full of flavour and surprisingly easy to make. It's perfect with prawns added, too.

1 tbsp sunflower oil
1 tbsp finely chopped root ginger
2 garlic cloves, finely chopped
1 small red chilli, finely chopped
1 lemon grass stalk, bruised
400ml vegetable or chicken stock
200ml coconut milk
1 large carrot, thinly sliced on the
   diagonal (160g)
handful of baby sweetcorn, halved
   lengthways, and further cut into
   2cm pieces if you want (80g)
160g chestnut mushrooms, cut into
   small pieces
1 red pepper, cut in 1cm pieces (160g)
3 large spring onions, cut in 1cm
   pieces (80g)
80g water chestnuts
handful of sugar snap peas, halved (80g)
sea salt and freshly ground black pepper
juice of ½ lime
Thai holy basil leaves, or coriander,
   to serve
prawn crackers, to serve

5 OF YOUR 5-A-DAY

Heat the oil in a large heavy-based saucepan and add the ginger, garlic, chilli and lemon grass. Fry over a medium heat for five minutes, stirring regularly, without colouring. Pour in the stock and coconut milk and cook gently for five minutes.

Add the carrot and baby sweetcorn and simmer for five minutes before adding the mushrooms and cooking for a further five minutes. Remove the lemon grass.

Add the red pepper, spring onions, water chestnuts and sugar snap peas. Cook for a final 10 minutes.

Add ¼ tsp salt and some pepper to taste. Finish with the lime juice. Sprinkle with the herbs. Serve with prawn crackers.

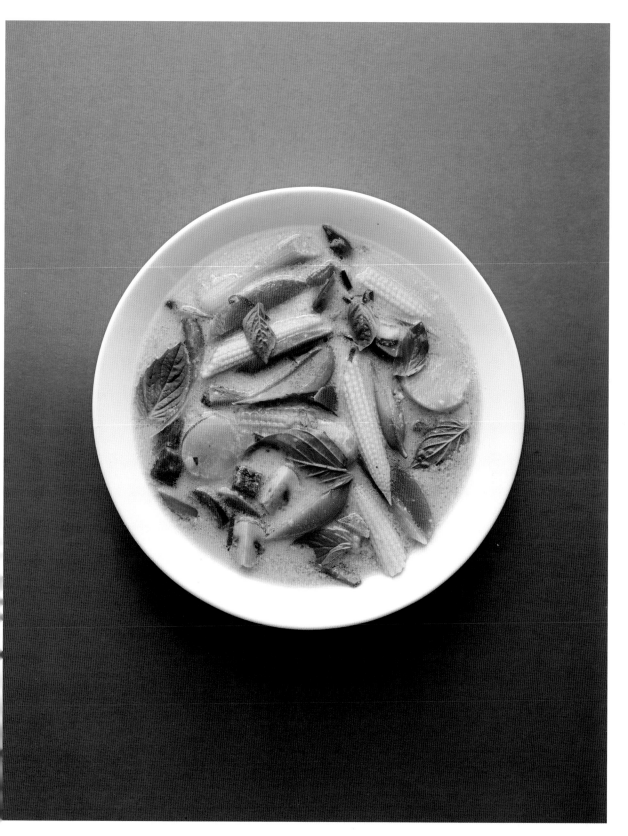

5 SPICY

Whether you prefer the robust heat of the Indian subcontinent or the more fragrant, aromatic flavours of South East Asia, there are plenty of recipes in this chapter which will spice up a whole host of different vegetables. If you like to cook your curries from scratch, authentic spices from all over the world are easily found at specialist retailers. However, if you prefer to take a shortcut, try one of the many fantastic ready-made spice pastes available from good supermarkets.

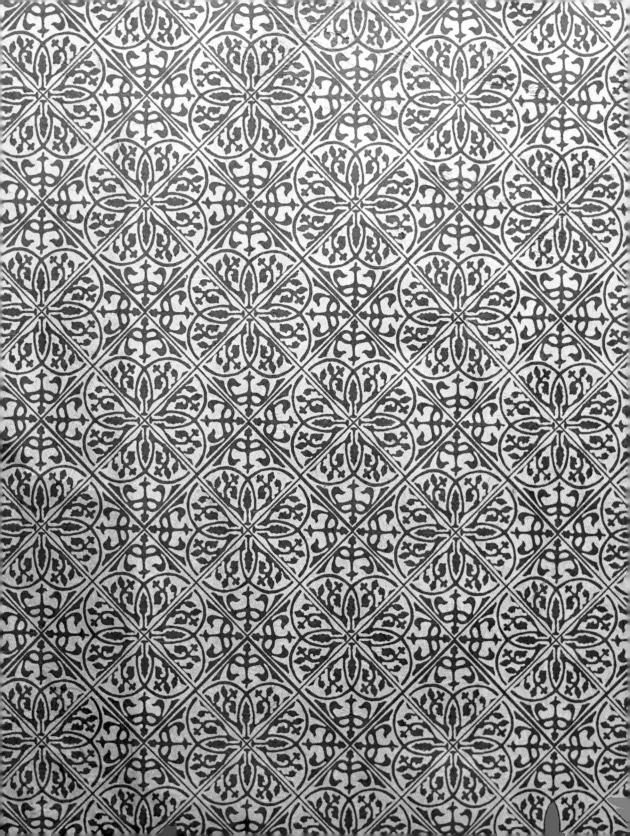

THAI GREEN CURRY | *serves 2*

Our five-a-day recipe adds roast butternut squash and red pepper to this dish for a variety of colours, textures and tastes. We use a very good ready-made Thai paste, so this dish is very easy to cook. It's perfect with chicken, too.

¼ butternut squash, cut into 1cm cubes (160g)
a little sunflower oil
1 medium onion, finely chopped (160g)
1 tbsp good-quality Thai green curry paste (we use Namjai)
120g chestnut mushrooms, cut into bite-sized pieces
handful of baby sweetcorn, halved (80g)
2 kaffir lime leaves
200ml coconut milk
200ml vegetable stock
80g canned bamboo shoots
80g green beans, halved
½ red pepper, cut into bite-sized pieces (80g)
large handful of spinach (about 40g)
handful of Thai holy basil, chopped (use regular basil if you can't find Thai, although it won't have the same authentic flavour), plus more to serve (optional)
½ tsp palm sugar, or to taste
juice of ½ lime, or to taste
½ tsp tamarind paste, or to taste
1 tbsp fish sauce (or soy sauce), or to taste

5 OF YOUR 5-A-DAY

Preheat the oven to 200°C/fan 180°C/400°F/gas mark 6. Roast the squash in a little oil for 20 minutes, or until just cooked (this will help to improve the flavour).

Fry the onion and curry paste in a little more oil for about five minutes, stirring constantly over a medium heat and adding 3 tbsp of water to ensure it doesn't burn. When the onion is soft, add the mushrooms and baby sweetcorn and fry for about two more minutes.

Add the kaffir lime leaves, coconut milk and stock and simmer for about 20 minutes. Add the bamboo shoots, green beans and red pepper and cook until the vegetables are just cooked but retain their crunch and colour. Remove the lime leaves and add the roasted squash.

Blitz the spinach with a little water in a small blender and add to the curry (this adds a nice vibrant green colour). Take off the heat and add the Thai holy basil. Taste and adjust the seasonings with palm sugar, lime juice, tamarind paste and fish sauce to balance the flavours to your taste. Serve sprinkled with more basil leaves, if you want.

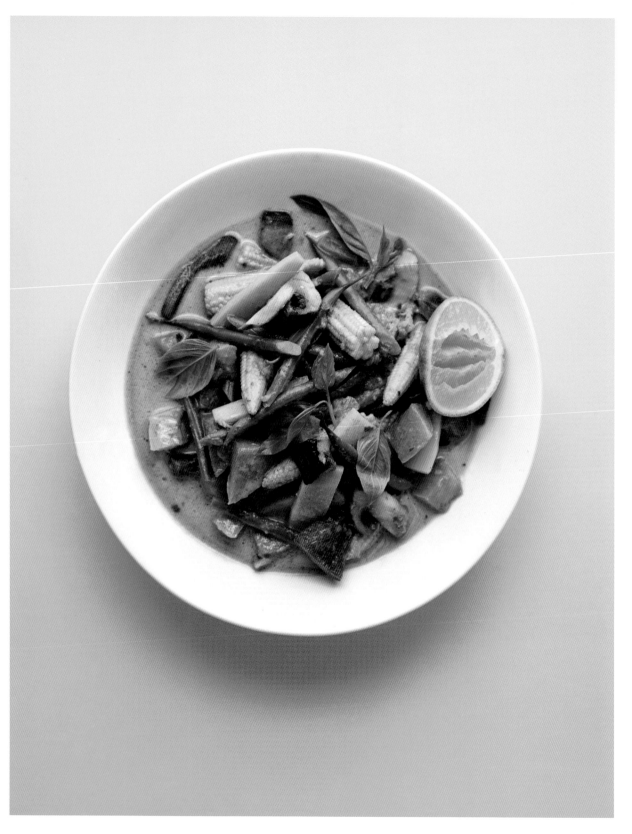

DAL WITH CHERRY TOMATOES, COURGETTE AND SPINACH | *serves 2*

Our dal is a light lentil recipe, influenced by the traditional dal tadka from Northern India. It is delicious with either rice or chapatis. The onion, garlic and chilli paste can be made in advance and frozen, or kept in the fridge for up to five days.

knob of root ginger (about 2cm cube)
1 garlic clove
1 red chilli
2 small celery sticks (80g)
1 small carrot (80g)
2 tbsp sunflower oil
1 cinnamon stick
2 bay leaves
a few fresh curry leaves (omit if you can't find fresh leaves, don't use dried)
1 tsp cumin seeds
1 tsp black mustard seeds
1 medium onion, finely chopped (160g)
90g red lentils (yields about 160g when cooked)
1 tsp ground coriander
½ tsp ground turmeric
pinch of chilli powder
small (230g) can of chopped tomatoes
1 courgette, cut into large bite-sized pieces (160g)
large handful of cherry tomatoes, halved (80g)
80g baby spinach
handful of coriander leaves
rice or chapatis, to serve

5 OF YOUR 5-A-DAY

Make a paste from the ginger, garlic and red chilli by blitzing in a small blender (or crushing in a mortar and pestle) and set aside. In the same blender, blitz the celery and carrot very finely with 2 tsp of water.

Heat the oil in a heavy-based saucepan and add the cinnamon stick and bay leaves, followed by the curry leaves, cumin and mustard seeds. Cook for 30 seconds, or until they start to change colour, but be careful not to burn them.

Add the onion and a little water to ensure the spices don't catch, then cook, stirring occasionally, until soft. Then add the garlic and carrot mixtures and cook for a further 15 minutes.

Meanwhile, rinse the lentils until the water runs clear. Add to boiling water in a separate pan and cook for 10 minutes or until tender. Drain and set aside.

Add the remaining dry spices to the onion mixture and cook for a couple more minutes before adding the canned tomatoes and drained lentils. Top up with hot water to your preferred consistency. Add the courgette and cook until just soft. Take off the heat and add the cherry tomatoes and spinach, which will cook in the residual heat. Stir in the coriander and serve with rice or chapatis.

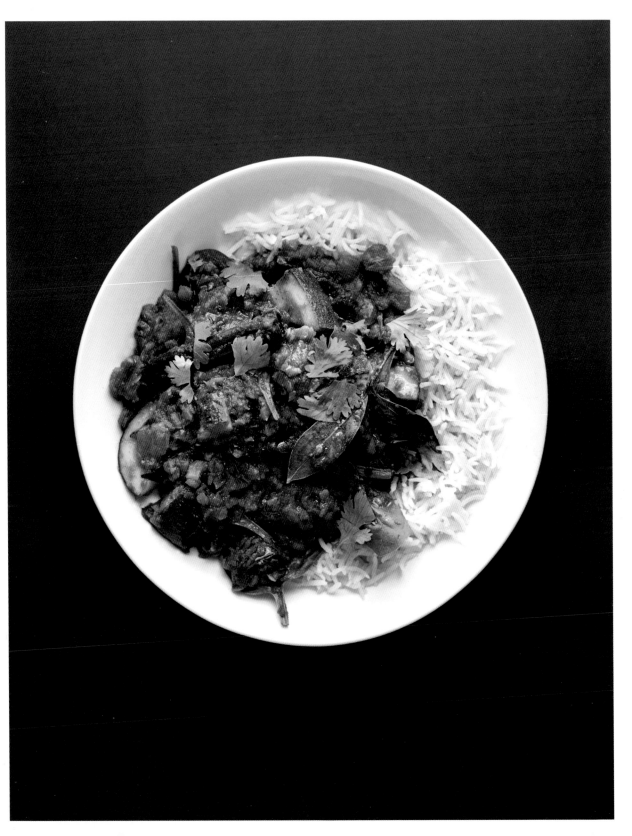

NORTH AFRICAN TAGINE WITH CAULIFLOWER 'COUSCOUS' | *serves 2*

The cauliflower couscous provides the real 'wow' factor here, and its subtle flavour is the perfect complement to this warmly spiced tagine. Toasted pumpkin seeds finish it all off with a healthy crunch.

160g sweet potato, cut into 2cm cubes (keep the skin on for a nutty flavour)
1 courgette, cut into 2cm cubes (160g)
2 tbsp olive oil
sea salt and freshly ground black pepper
1 medium onion, finely chopped (160g)
2 tsp ras-el-hanout
2 handfuls of cherry tomatoes, halved (160g)
400g can of chickpeas, drained and rinsed (net weight 240g)
10g sultanas
10g dried apricots
10g pumpkin seeds
10g flaked almonds
small head of cauliflower, florets only (160g)
small handful of mint leaves, finely chopped
small handful of coriander leaves, finely chopped

5 OF YOUR 5-A-DAY

Preheat the oven to 200°C/fan 180°C/400°F/gas mark 6.

Place the sweet potato and courgette in a roasting tray with 1 tbsp of the oil and plenty of seasoning and roast for 20–25 minutes until soft.

Meanwhile, fry the onion in the remaining 1 tbsp of oil for about 10 minutes until soft and golden. Add the ras-el-hanout and cook for two minutes over a medium heat, stirring continuously and adding a little water if the spices look like they are catching.

Add the tomatoes, chickpeas, sultanas and apricots. Pour in 300ml of water, bring to a simmer, cover and cook for 30 minutes, stirring occasionally, until the tagine is flavourful and rich. Stir in the roasted vegetables and continue to cook for a further five to 10 minutes.

Toast the pumpkin seeds and flaked almonds in a dry pan until lightly golden. Set aside.

Put the cauliflower florets in a food processor and pulse for a few moments until you get the consistency of couscous. Put in a microwaveable bowl with 1 tbsp of water and a sprinkling of salt, cover with cling film and microwave for about five minutes until cooked.

When ready to serve, mix the herbs into the cauliflower 'couscous' and ladle the tagine on top. Top with the pumpkin seeds and flaked almonds.

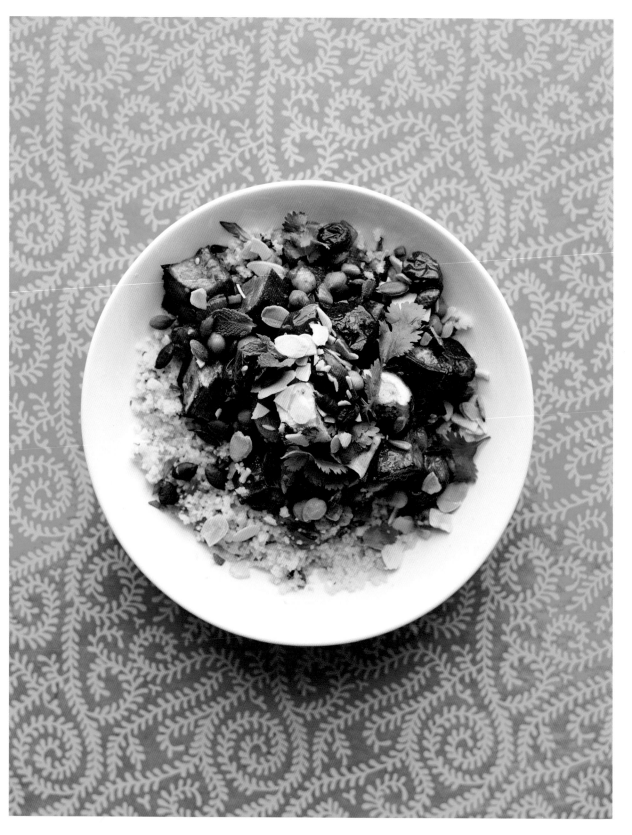

SMOKY CHIPOTLE CHILLI | *serves 2*

This wholesome chilli is made with chipotle, a specific type of jalapeño often used in Mexican cuisine. They are picked when red and very ripe, then smoked. They give this chilli a wonderfully distinctive, smoky, earthy flavour.

1 chipotle chilli, or 1–2 tsp chipotle paste
60g dried aduki beans, or 120g (drained weight) canned aduki beans, with the liquid from the can
2 tbsp sunflower oil
sea salt and freshly ground black pepper
1 large red onion, chopped (160g)
2 garlic cloves, finely chopped
2 small celery sticks, finely chopped (80g)
½ red pepper, finely chopped (80g)
160g mushrooms, cut into small pieces
1 tsp ground cumin
1 tsp dried oregano
¼ tsp hot chilli powder, or to taste
1 tbsp tomato purée
1 tbsp plain flour
1 large ripe tomato, finely chopped
½ x 400g can of kidney or cannellini beans
1 tsp Worcestershire sauce, or to taste
½ tsp caster sugar, or to taste
rice or baked potatoes, to serve

If using the dried chilli, soak it in a mug in a small amount of warm water to cover for 20 minutes until soft. Reserving the soaking liquid, remove the chilli and finely chop.

Meanwhile, if you are using dried aduki beans, cook them according to the packet instructions (but you might need to cook them for a little longer as you want them nice and soft). Drain and reserve the cooking water. Mash the cooked or canned beans lightly with a little of the oil, seasoning with salt and pepper.

Heat the remaining oil in a heavy-based saucepan and fry the onion for about five minutes until soft. Add the garlic, celery and red pepper and fry for a further eight minutes until soft and lightly coloured. Add the mushrooms with the cumin, oregano, chilli powder and finely chopped chipotle plus its soaking liquid, or the chipotle paste. Continue cooking for five to eight minutes.

Add the tomato purée and cook for another two minutes before adding the flour. Cook for two minutes more before adding the tomato, aduki beans and kidney beans. Add enough of the aduki bean canning or cooking liquid to make a good consistency. Taste and add the Worcestershire sauce and sugar. Season, then cover and cook, stirring occasionally, for about 45 minutes. Serve with rice or baked potatoes.

5 OF YOUR
5-A-DAY

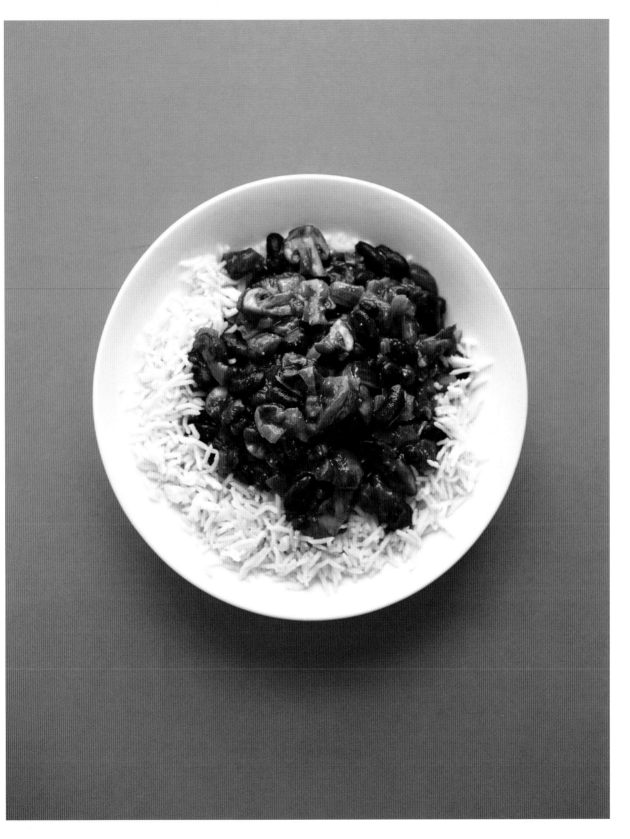

QUICK CHICKPEA, MUSHROOM AND SPINACH CURRY | *serves 2*

This little marvel can be knocked up in not much more than 15 minutes from storecupboard ingredients while waiting for the rice to cook, so it is super-convenient. It includes many of our five-a-day staples: onions, tomato purée, spinach, mushrooms and canned chickpeas.

1 medium onion, finely chopped (160g)
1 garlic clove, finely chopped
a little sunflower oil
1–2 tbsp hot madras curry powder or a
*   similar curry paste*
2 tbsp tomato purée
160g mushrooms, cut into
*   bite-sized pieces*
400g can of chickpeas, with the liquid
*   from the can*
160g spinach
1 tsp garam masala
a few coriander leaves (optional)
1 tbsp natural yogurt (optional)
rice or chapatis, to serve

**5 OF YOUR
5-A-DAY**

Fry the onion and garlic in the oil until soft. Add the curry powder or paste and fry for about one minute over a high heat, stirring continuously, until the spices have cooked.

Add the tomato purée and mushrooms and cook for a further couple of minutes before adding the chickpeas and their liquid. Top up with a little more hot water if you think it's needed and cook for about 15 minutes.

Stir in the spinach until wilted and sprinkle over the garam masala and a few coriander leaves, if using. Stir in the yogurt, if you prefer a creamier curry. Serve with rice or chapatis.

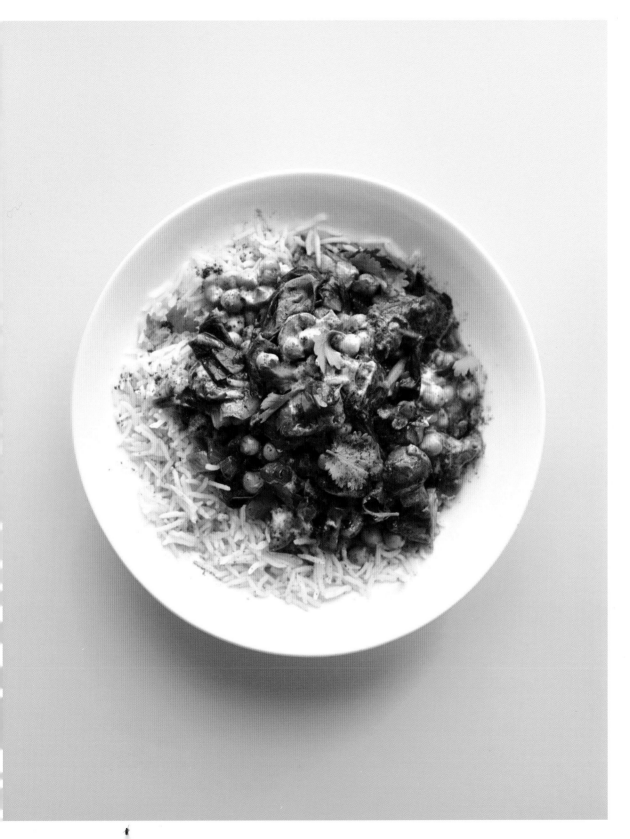

GOAN AUBERGINE CURRY WITH
COCONUT AND TAMARIND | *serves 2*

A tangy, mildly spiced curry with ginger and coconut. This dish is traditionally made with fish or seafood; either will complement our colourful vegetable version.

For the paste

2 garlic cloves, finely chopped
2 tsp finely chopped root ginger
1 green chilli, finely chopped
4 black peppercorns
2 tsp ground coriander
2 tsp ground cumin
1 tsp fennel seeds
1 tsp ground turmeric

For the vegetables

2 tbsp vegetable oil, plus more if needed
1 cinnamon stick
2 bay leaves
1 medium onion, finely chopped (160g)
2–3 large tomatoes, chopped (160g)
160g sweet potato, cut into bite-sized
   pieces
small aubergine, cut into bite-sized
   pieces (160g)
40g fresh grated coconut (or frozen/
   desiccated coconut), plus more
   to taste (optional)
300ml vegetable stock
handful of green beans, halved (80g)
80g frozen peas, defrosted
sea salt
½ tsp tamarind paste
large handful of coriander,
   finely chopped

**5 OF YOUR
5-A-DAY**

To make the paste, blend all the ingredients with 2 tbsp of water in a small blender (or use a mortar and pestle).

Heat the oil in a heavy-based saucepan and fry the cinnamon and bay leaves for a minute or so. Add the onion and cook for about eight minutes until golden brown. Then add the curry paste, you may need to add a little more oil. Fry the curry paste for five minutes, then add the tomatoes followed by the sweet potato and aubergine. Add the coconut and pour in the stock. Cover and cook for 25 minutes, until the vegetables are tender, adding the green beans for the final 10 minutes.

Add the peas and a little more water or coconut depending on how thick you like your curry. Take out the cinnamon stick and bay leaves.

Taste and season with salt and the tamarind, then scatter over the coriander to serve.

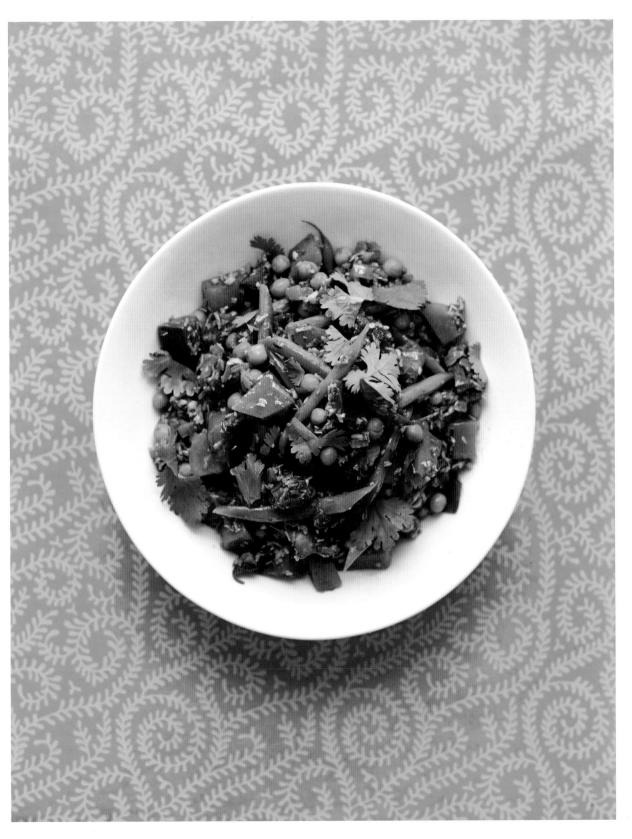

INDIAN-SPICED VEGETABLES | *serves 2*

This versatile recipe uses classic Indian flavourings to spice up any combination of vegetables. Great as a wholesome vegan or vegetarian dish or as a side with beef, chicken or prawns.

2 tbsp sunflower oil
1 tsp cumin seeds
1 tsp mustard seeds
2 tsp finely chopped root ginger
1 garlic clove, finely chopped
1 medium onion, sliced (160g)
1 green chilli, whole but slit
1 small cauliflower, broken into small
   florets (160g)
1 medium carrot, sliced on the
   diagonal (80g)
handful of green beans, halved (80g)
½ tsp sea salt
1 red pepper, cut into bite-sized
   pieces (160g)
½ tsp ground ginger
½ tsp ground turmeric
½ tsp chilli powder
1 tsp ground coriander
½ tsp ground cumin
2 large handfuls of cherry tomatoes,
   halved (160g)
1 tbsp lemon juice
large handful of coriander,
   roughly chopped

**5 OF YOUR
5-A-DAY**

Heat the oil in a heavy-based saucepan, add the cumin and mustard seeds and cook for 30 seconds until the seeds start to change colour and pop.

Add the ginger and garlic and fry for a further 30 seconds before adding the onion and chilli. Fry for two minutes before mixing in the cauliflower, carrot and green beans. Add the salt and cook for about five minutes, stirring occasionally. Add the pepper and cook for five minutes until the vegetables are tender but still retain a crunch.

Add the ground spices and cook for two minutes before adding the tomatoes. Cook everything for about five minutes, until the tomatoes have broken down. Remove the chilli and finish with the lemon juice and coriander.

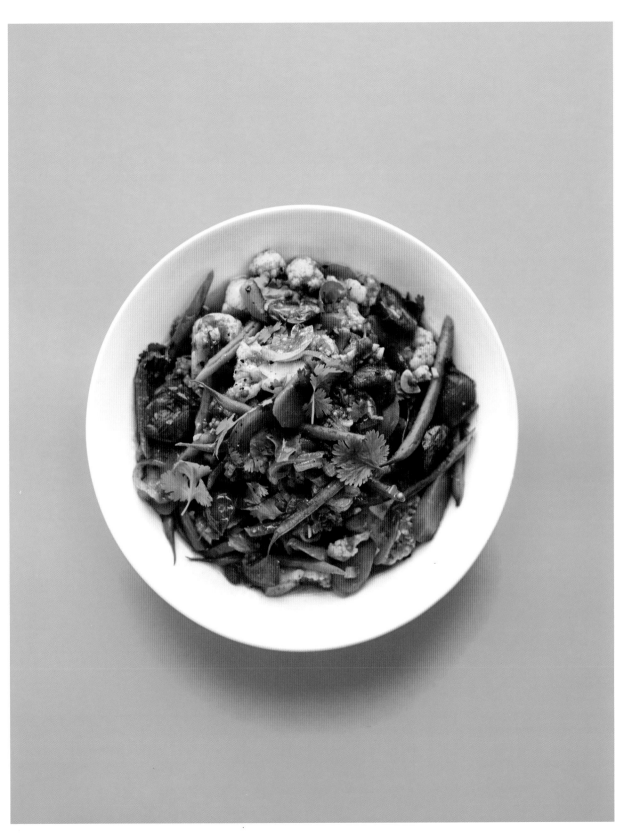

CARIBBEAN PUMPKIN AND PEA CURRY | *serves 2*

A classic coconut curry from the West Indies. Our version uses the humble British green pea to good effect. Its bright green colour, combined with the radiant orange pumpkin and mango, reminds us of the lush Caribbean landscape.

2 tbsp sunflower oil
1 onion, finely chopped (160g)
1 scotch bonnet pepper, kept whole
2 tsp finely chopped root ginger
2 garlic cloves, finely chopped
1 heaped tbsp mild madras
   curry powder
1 tsp ground allspice
½ tsp ground turmeric
2 large tomatoes, finely chopped (160g)
400ml can of coconut milk
sea salt
¼ pumpkin or butternut squash, cut into
   bite-sized pieces (160g)
400g can of gungo peas, black-eyed
   beans or chickpeas, with the liquid
   from the can
½ red pepper, finely chopped (80g)
½ tsp Worcestershire sauce
40g frozen peas, defrosted
½ mango, chopped (80g)
2 tsp hot pepper sauce

5 OF YOUR 5-A-DAY

Heat the oil in a heavy-based saucepan and fry the onion for five to eight minutes until light golden. Make a slit in the scotch bonnet and add to the pan whole with the ginger and garlic. Fry for a further two minutes.

Add a splash of water before adding the curry powder, allspice and turmeric. Fry for a further two minutes before adding the tomatoes and a little more water if the spices threaten to catch on the base of the pan.

Pour in the coconut milk and ½ tsp salt before adding the squash. Tip in the gungo peas and their liquid and bring slowly up to the boil. Immediately reduce the heat and simmer gently, uncovered, for 20 minutes, until the squash is cooked. Taste, and if your curry has reached the desired heat, remove the scotch bonnet, otherwise leave in if you prefer a hotter curry. Add the pepper and Worcestershire sauce and cook for a further three minutes.

Just before serving, stir in the peas and mango and cook for two minutes before seasoning with more salt (if needed) and the hot pepper sauce.

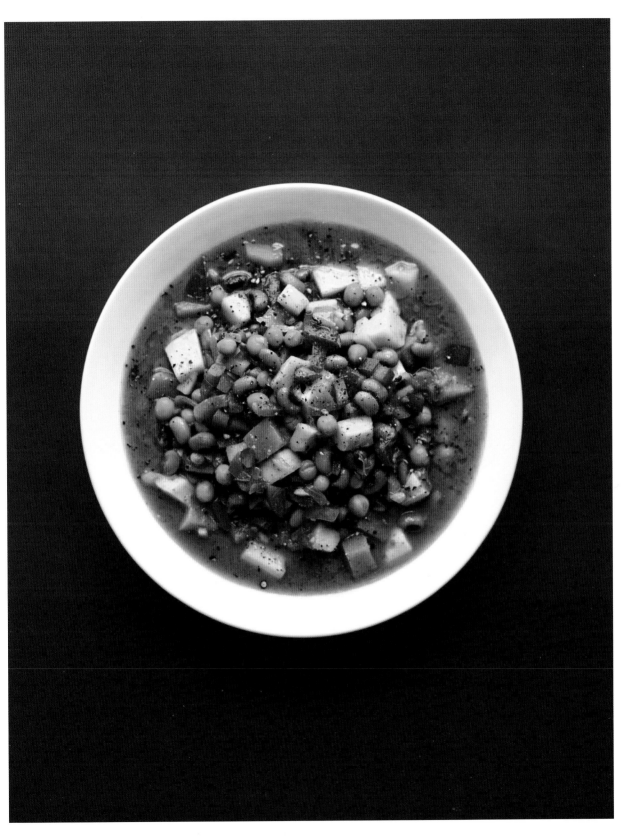

SRI LANKAN SQUASH AND CAULIFLOWER CURRY | *serves 2*

Sri Lanka's cuisine is heavily influenced by that of its neighbour, southern India. Our recipe uses tamarind, a traditional souring ingredient, to give a delicious sweet and sour flavour.

2 tbsp vegetable oil
6 cloves
6 green cardamom pods
2 tsp black mustard seeds
small handful of kaffir lime leaves
1 large red onion, finely chopped (160g)
4 garlic cloves, finely chopped
1 tbsp finely chopped root ginger
1 red or green chilli, finely chopped
½ tsp ground turmeric
2–3 large tomatoes, chopped (160g), or
    ½ x 400g can of chopped tomatoes
¼ butternut squash or pumpkin, peeled
    and cut into large pieces (160g)
small aubergine, cut into bite-sized
    pieces (160g)
300ml vegetable stock
100g creamed coconut
1 small cauliflower, broken into small
    florets (160g)
1 tsp tamarind paste
1 tsp palm sugar
1 tsp lime juice
dash of soy sauce
sea salt
1 tsp garam masala
2 tbsp natural yogurt sprinkled with
    cinnamon (optional)
rice or chapatis, to serve

5 OF YOUR 5-A-DAY

To make the sauce, heat the oil in a heavy-based saucepan and fry the cloves and green cardamom followed by the mustard seeds and lime leaves. When the mustard seeds start to pop (about 30 seconds), add the onion and fry for eight minutes until golden brown.

Add the garlic, ginger, chilli and turmeric and cook for a further three minutes, stirring continuously and adding a little water if necessary to stop the onions and spices catching.

Add the tomatoes, butternut squash, aubergine, 200ml of the stock and the creamed coconut and simmer with a lid on for 15 minutes. Then add the cauliflower, remaining stock, tamarind, palm sugar, lime juice, soy sauce, salt and garam masala. Cook for another 15 minutes, uncovered, until all the vegetables are soft.

Serve with the cinnamon yogurt (if using) and some rice or chapatis.

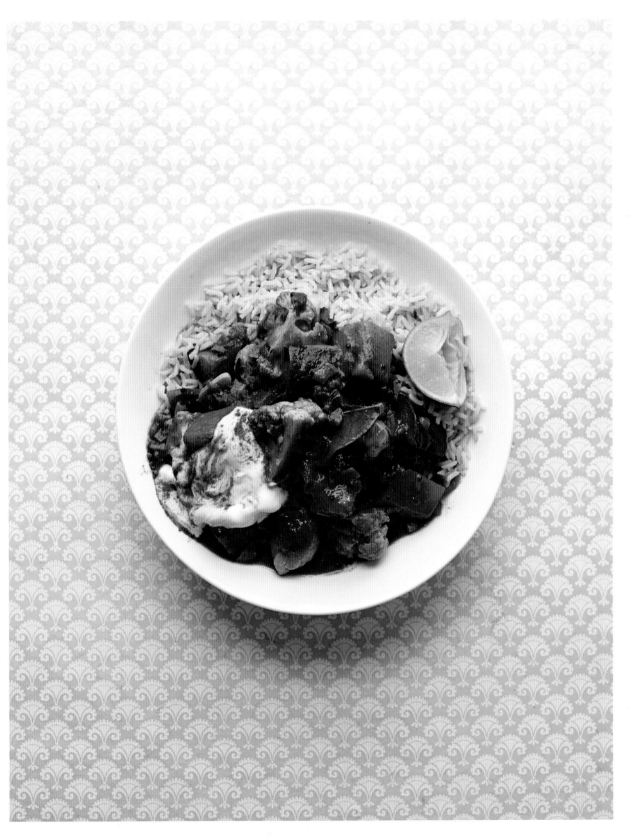

MASSAMAN CURRY
WITH SWEET POTATO | *serves 2*

A mildly spiced Thai dish with Malaysian influences, this is a rich, colourful alternative to a Thai green curry. We use a great massaman curry paste, so this is very easy to make (it also works brilliantly with beef). For a hotter curry, just add more paste or include some chopped red chillies.

2 tbsp vegetable oil
2 tbsp massaman curry paste (we use Thai Taste brand)
1 large red onion, chopped (160g)
160g sweet potato, cut into 2cm cubes
160g chestnut mushrooms, cut into bite-sized pieces
1 red pepper, chopped (160g)
small aubergine, cut into 2cm cubes (160g)
300ml vegetable stock
50g creamed coconut
juice of ½ lime, or to taste
1 tsp palm sugar, or to taste
a few leaves of Thai holy basil

**5 OF YOUR
5-A-DAY**

Heat the oil in a heavy-based saucepan and fry the curry paste, stirring constantly, for about one minute. Add the onion, sweet potato and 3 tbsp of water and fry for another five minutes, stirring constantly.

Add the rest of the vegetables and make sure everything is coated with the curry paste.

Pour in the stock and simmer, uncovered, for about 25 minutes until all the vegetables are cooked. Add the creamed coconut and season with the lime juice and palm sugar to taste.

Take off the heat and serve with a small sprinkling of chopped Thai holy basil, but not too much as you don't want the herb to overpower the dish.

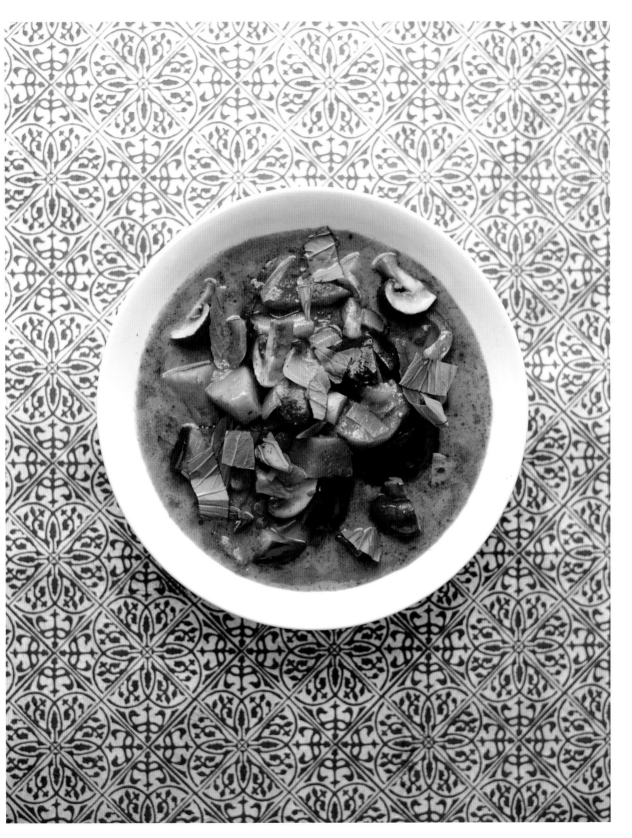

PERFECT PILAU | *serves 2*

A wholesome and spicy rice dish with a West Indian influence.
This recipe uses brown rice, which takes a little longer to cook
than white but is better for you. It is made in one pot to allow
all the different flavours to integrate.

2 tbsp sunflower oil
1 medium onion, chopped (160g)
80g mushrooms, cut into bite-sized
  pieces
1 courgette, chopped into bite-sized
  pieces (160g)
½ red pepper, chopped into bite-sized
  pieces (80g)
2 tsp ground cumin
2 tsp ground coriander
¼ tsp chilli powder (optional)
400g can of chopped tomatoes
400g can of gungo peas or kidney
  beans, drained and rinsed
  (net weight 240g)
1 tbsp tomato ketchup
2 tsp hot pepper sauce
2 tbsp soy sauce
1 tsp Worcestershire sauce
2 tbsp coconut milk (optional)
1 tsp garam masala
100g brown long-grain rice
300ml vegetable stock

5 OF YOUR
5-A-DAY

Heat the oil in a heavy-based saucepan and fry the onion until light golden brown. Add the mushrooms, courgette and red pepper and fry for about 10 minutes.

Add the cumin, coriander and chilli powder (if using) and continue to fry for about three minutes until the spices have cooked. Pour in the tomatoes and cook over a high heat for about five minutes.

Tip in the gungo peas or kidney beans followed by the ketchup, hot pepper sauce, soy sauce, Worcestershire sauce, coconut milk (if using) and garam masala.

Add the rice and the stock, give it a stir and, when it is bubbling vigorously, cover and reduce the heat to its lowest setting. Cook for about 40 minutes, or until the rice is tender.

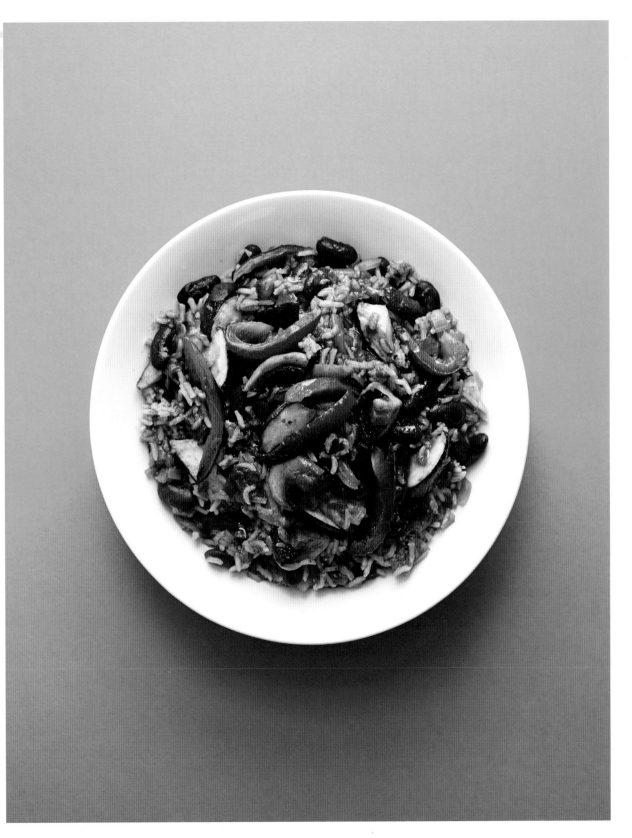

STIR-FRIED ORIENTAL NOODLES WITH GINGER AND SESAME | *serves 2*

A colourful combination of many different vegetables, ideal for lunch or a light supper, and just as good without the noodles if you want to cut the carbs. Add prawns or chicken, if you want.

1 tbsp sesame seeds
2 tbsp sunflower oil
1 garlic clove, finely chopped
2 tbsp finely chopped root ginger
4 large spring onions, sliced on the diagonal (80g)
2 tsp finely chopped red chilli
handful of baby sweetcorn, halved lengthways (80g)
160g mushrooms, sliced
1 large carrot, halved lengthways and thinly sliced on the diagonal (160g)
handful of broccoli florets (80g)
½ red pepper, sliced (80g)
sea salt and freshly ground black pepper
1 head of pak choi, stems thinly sliced, leaves roughly chopped (80g)
handful of sugar snap peas, halved lengthways (80g)
50g fresh egg noodles
1 tbsp rice vinegar
2 tbsp dark soy sauce
2 tsp sesame oil
juice of 1 lime
½ tsp honey (optional)

5 OF YOUR 5-A-DAY

In a small frying pan, dry-roast the sesame seeds until they turn golden brown. Take off the heat and set aside.

Heat the sunflower oil in a wok and fry the garlic and ginger for about one minute until lightly coloured but not burning. Add the spring onions and red chilli and cook for a further two minutes before adding the baby sweetcorn, mushrooms, carrot, broccoli and red pepper. Season and continue to stir-fry for four or five minutes.

Add the pak choi stems followed by the sugar snap peas and, after two minutes, add the pak choi leaves and the noodles. Cook for a further two minutes, until the noodles have warmed through.

Lastly, add the rice vinegar, soy sauce, sesame oil, lime juice and honey (if using), give everything a toss and serve sprinkled with the toasted sesame seeds.

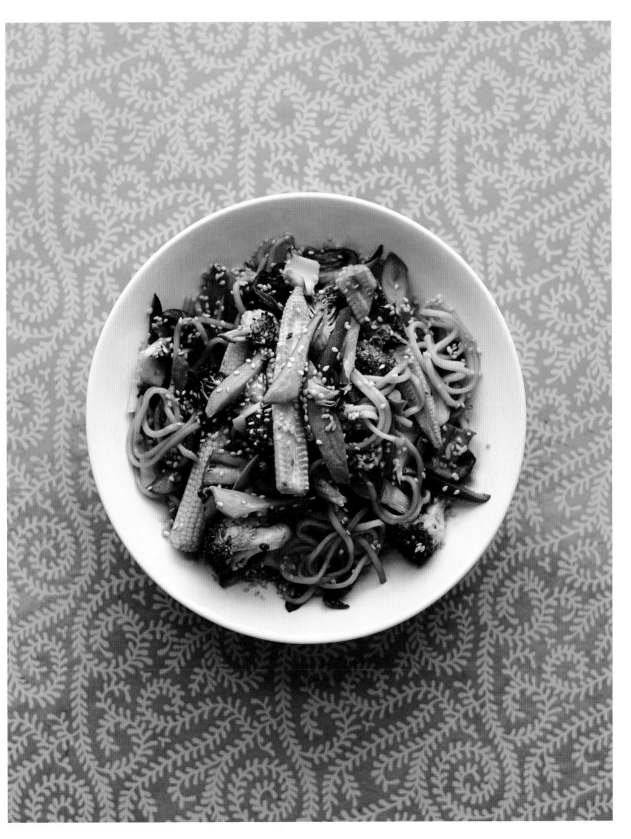

PEANUT SPICED VEGETABLES | *serves 2*

Peanut sauce is used widely in cuisine across Asia and Africa and its rich and distinctive flavour complements all kinds of vegetables. This stir-fry is big on taste and quick to make. You can use any combination of vegetables: greens or kale work well as alternatives.

For the sauce
1 tbsp groundnut oil
1 tbsp oyster sauce
1 tbsp kecap manis
1 tbsp soy sauce
1 tsp rice vinegar
1 tbsp smooth peanut butter
1 tbsp finely chopped coriander leaves

For the vegetables
1 tbsp peanuts
1 tbsp sunflower oil
2 tsp finely chopped root ginger
1 garlic clove, finely chopped
2 tsp finely chopped red chilli
1 small onion, finely sliced (80g)
½ head of broccoli, cut into small
   pieces (160g)
handful of green beans, topped and
   tailed (80g)
large handful of baby sweetcorn, halved
   lengthways (80g)
1 red pepper, sliced (160g)
5 asparagus spears, chopped (80g)
1 head of pak choi, stems finely
   chopped, leaves shredded (80g)
handful of mange tout (80g)

5 OF YOUR
5-A-DAY

Combine all the sauce ingredients together with 4 tbsp of water and set aside.

Place the peanuts in a dry pan and toast until golden brown. Set these aside, too.

Heat the sunflower oil in a wok and fry the ginger, garlic and chilli for two minutes, then follow with the onion, broccoli and green beans, cooking for five minutes. Add the sweetcorn, red pepper and asparagus and stir-fry for a further five minutes.

Add the pak choi stems and cook for a minute before adding the mange tout and pak choi leaves.

Stir in the sauce, heat through for one minute, then take off the heat and serve with the toasted peanuts on top.

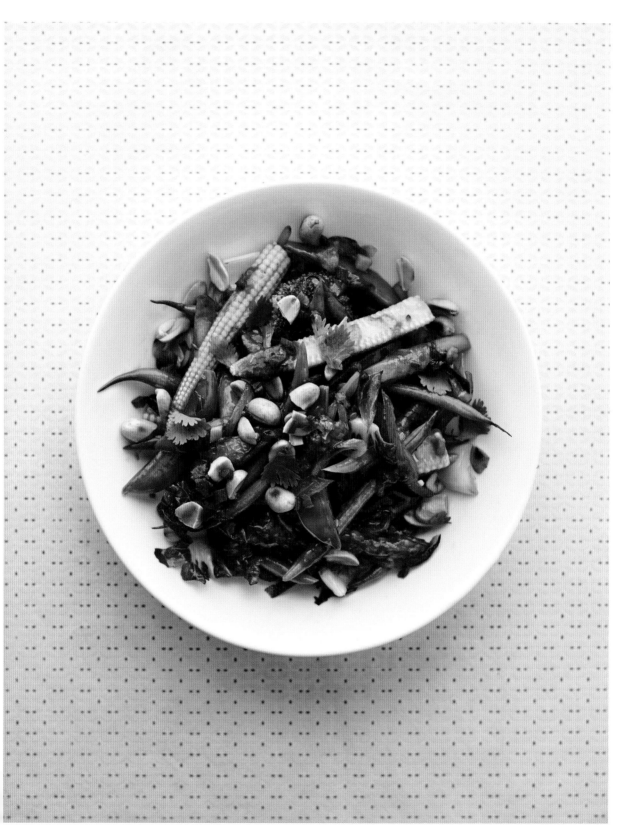

AFGHANI-STYLE STEW WITH MINT AND PINE NUTS | *serves 2*

A delicious, hearty, mildly spiced stew. The traditional ingredients of spinach, pine nuts and yogurt are a really interesting combination, while the addition of mint makes this a great dish to accompany lamb.

2 tbsp vegetable oil
1 tsp cumin seeds
1 medium onion, finely chopped (160g)
3 garlic cloves, finely chopped
1 tbsp finely chopped root ginger
1 red chilli, finely chopped
1 tsp ground coriander
1½ tsp ground cumin
½ tsp ground turmeric
½ tsp ground cinnamon
¼ tsp freshly grated nutmeg
small (230g) can of chopped tomatoes
small aubergine, cut into cubes (160g)
400g can of chickpeas, drained and
    rinsed (net weight 240g)
2 tsp finely grated unwaxed lemon zest
2 tbsp pine nuts, toasted (see page 38,
    following method for peanuts)
2 tbsp raisins
2 tbsp natural yogurt
2 tsp garam masala
160g spinach, roughly chopped
sea salt
3 tbsp finely chopped
    mint leaves

5 OF YOUR 5-A-DAY

Heat the oil in a heavy-based saucepan and fry the cumin seeds for 30 seconds before adding the onion. Fry for a further five minutes until light golden.

Add the garlic, ginger and chilli and fry for a further three minutes, adding 2 tbsp of water to stop the mixture catching on the pan.

Add the ground coriander, cumin, turmeric, cinnamon and nutmeg and cook for two minutes. Add the tomatoes, aubergine, chickpeas, lemon zest, pine nuts and raisins, then pour in 400ml of hot water. Cover and simmer for 15 minutes.

When the aubergine is cooked, add the yogurt and garam masala. Add the spinach and stir in for one minute to wilt.

Season with salt and serve sprinkled with the mint.

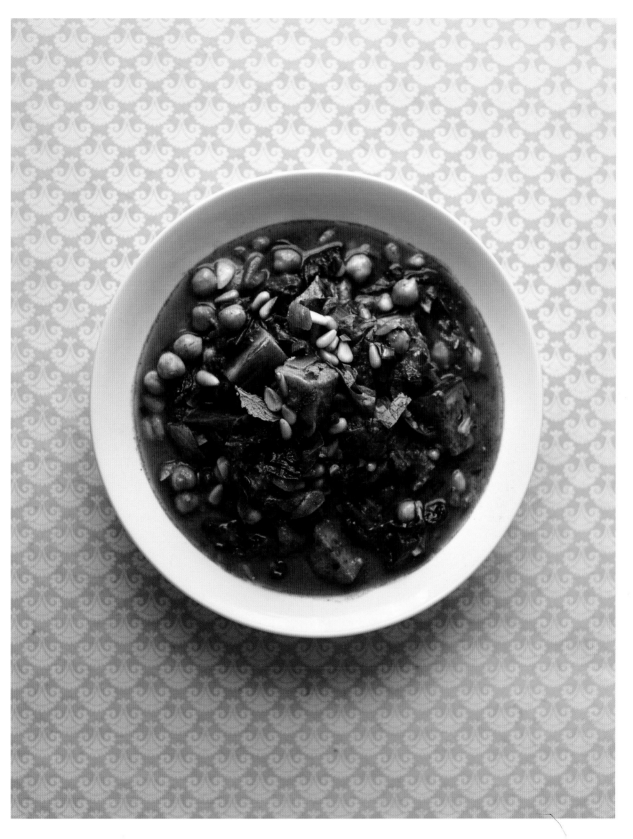

NASI GORENG | *serves 2*

Traditionally this Indonesian stir-fried dish is made with leftover rice, but we use cauliflower 'rice' instead. This makes the dish lighter and lower in carbohydrate as well as providing an additional portion of your five-a-day. A very quick stir-fry to make, this works well with chicken, prawns and our Chilli sambal (see page 176) if you like it hot.

1 cauliflower, florets only (160g)
2 tbsp groundnut oil
1 medium onion, finely chopped (160g)
2 garlic cloves, finely chopped
1 tsp finely chopped root ginger
2 red chillies, finely chopped
2 eggs, lightly beaten
pinch of sea salt
1 small leek, trimmed and sliced (80g)
160g chestnut mushrooms, quartered
1 red pepper, finely chopped (160g)
large handful of beansprouts (80g)
1 tbsp dark soy sauce
sea salt and freshly ground
    black pepper

Make the cauliflower 'rice': place the florets in a food processor and blitz until you have the consistency of rice.

Heat 1 tbsp of the oil in a wok and add the onion, garlic, ginger and chillies. Stir-fry for two minutes, then add the cauliflower 'rice' and continue to fry for three to four minutes.

Make a well in the cauliflower mixture, add the eggs and salt and stir for two to three minutes until the eggs are cooked. Remove the mixture and set aside, keeping it warm, but don't clean the wok.

Heat the remaining 1 tbsp of oil in the wok and add the leek. Stir-fry for two minutes before adding the mushrooms and pepper. Stir-fry for a further five to seven minutes.

To finish, add the beansprouts, the cauliflower mixture and soy sauce. Season to taste and serve immediately.

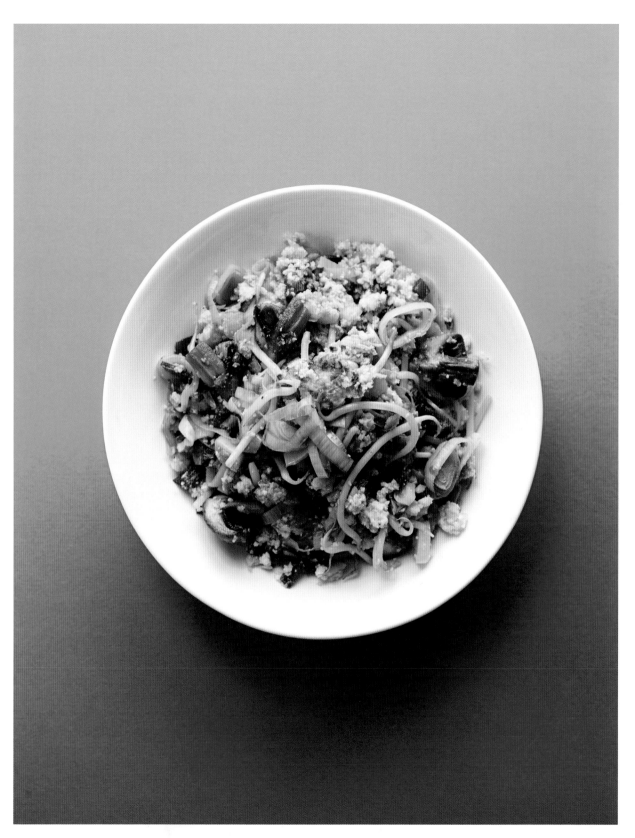

EVERYDAY 5

Getting your five-a-day every day in a way that suits the whole family – particularly the kids – is not easy. But gradually introducing new varieties of vegetables and slowly increasing the amount on offer is a sure way to get everyone eating more. In this chapter we have taken a range of traditional family favourites and adapted them to include more vegetables. Tried and tested many times on our own families, they don't even notice the absence of meat.

'FIVE' PASTA SAUCE | *serves 2*

*Sometimes the simplest ideas are the best. This rich tomato
and mushroom pasta sauce contains no unusual ingredients
but packs in all your five-a-day in a very unassuming way.
Add meatballs, if you want.*

2 tbsp olive oil
1 medium onion, very finely
    chopped (160g)
2 garlic cloves, crushed
1 medium carrot, very finely
    chopped (80g)
2 small celery sticks, very finely
    chopped (80g)
1 small leek, trimmed and very finely
    sliced (80g)
1 red pepper, very finely chopped (160g)
160g mushrooms, sliced
1 tsp sea salt
10g tomato purée
1 tbsp plain flour
4 tbsp red wine
230g can of chopped tomatoes
½ tsp caster sugar
bouquet garni of basil stalks, parsley
    stalks, bay leaf, sprigs of thyme

To serve
30g Parmesan cheese, shaved or
    finely grated
a few basil leaves
pasta

Heat the oil in a heavy-based saucepan and fry the onion
for about 10 minutes until soft. Add the garlic and cook for
a further two minutes before adding the carrot, celery, leek,
pepper, mushrooms and salt. Cook for a further 10 minutes
until the vegetables are soft.

Add the tomato purée and cook for one minute before adding
the flour. Stir for two minutes before adding the red wine.
When the wine has evaporated, add the tomatoes, sugar
and bouquet garni and pour in 150ml of water. Bring to the
boil, then reduce the heat to a simmer and cook for about
40 minutes until reduced, rich and flavourful.

Remove the bouquet garni and serve with your pasta of
choice, sprinkled with the Parmesan and basil.

5 OF YOUR
5-A-DAY

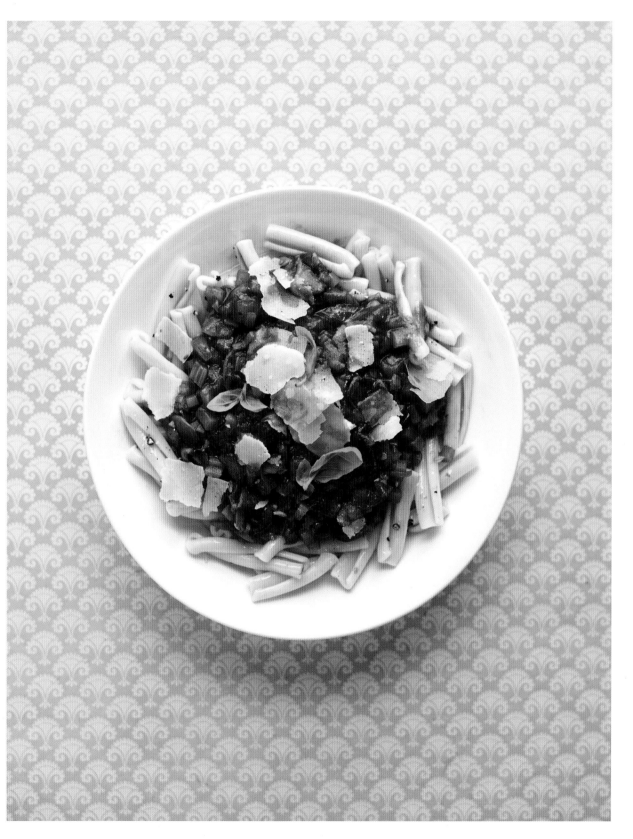

PISTO CON HUEVOS | *serves 2*

A rustic Spanish classic, very much like ratatouille but served with an egg on top. Our recipe is very versatile and could be made with a variety of vegetables. Dip crusty bread into the soft eggs and mop up the garlicky vegetables for a great lunch or light supper. This is also lovely with ham.

2 tbsp olive oil
1 large red onion, finely chopped (160g)
4 garlic cloves, finely chopped
1 red chilli, finely chopped (optional)
small aubergine, cut into bite-sized
  pieces (160g)
1 red pepper, cut into bite-sized
  pieces (160g)
1 courgette, cut into bite-sized
  pieces (160g)
2 tomatoes, roughly chopped
sea salt and freshly ground black pepper
a few thyme leaves
1 tsp good-quality Spanish sweet
  paprika, plus more to serve
230g can of chopped tomatoes
handful of parsley leaves, chopped
2 eggs
20g Manchego cheese, finely grated
crusty bread, to serve

**5 OF YOUR
5-A-DAY**

Preheat the oven to 190°C/fan 170°C/375°F/gas mark 5.

Heat the oil in a heavy-based saucepan and fry the onion until soft. Add the garlic and chilli and continue cooking for a further two minutes before adding the rest of the vegetables. Season with salt, pepper, the thyme and paprika. Add the canned tomatoes and cook uncovered for 20–30 minutes until all the vegetables are soft and sweet.

Take off the heat and mix in the parsley (reserving a few leaves to serve). Spoon the pisto into an ovenproof dish and make two dips for the eggs. Crack the eggs into the hollows and bake in the oven for about 15 minutes, or until the whites have just set but the yolks are still runny.

Remove from the oven and sprinkle with the cheese, remaining parsley and a little paprika.

Serve with lots of crusty bread.

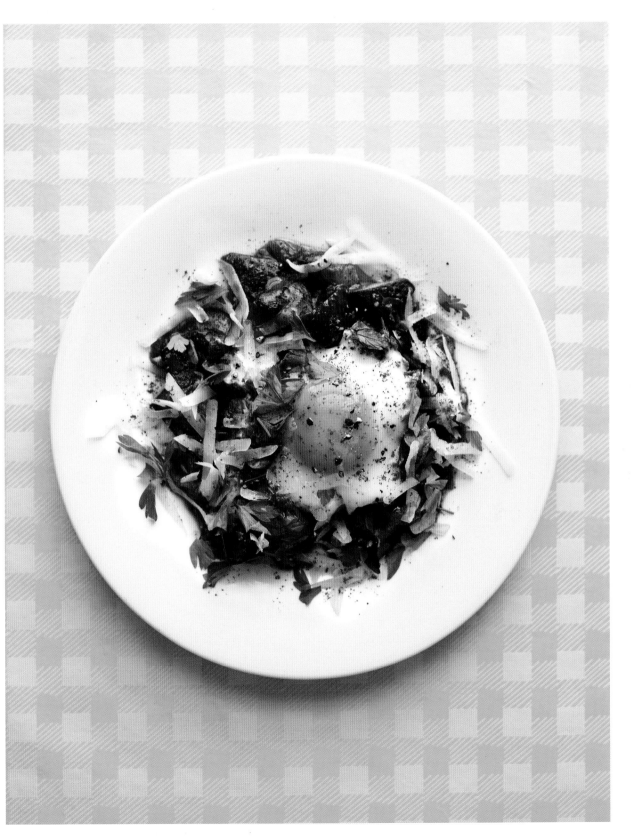

AUBERGINE PARMIGIANA | *serves 2*

A healthy vegetable bake based on the traditional Italian Parmigiana. Our version combines layered aubergines and courgettes with a thick tomato sauce. This is a really hearty, filling dish, perfect for sharing. Add mozzarella between the layers for a richer meal.

2 tbsp olive oil
1 tbsp green pesto
1 large aubergine, sliced into 1cm
   rounds (300g+)
1 large courgette, sliced 5mm-thick
   lengthways (160g+)
½ yellow pepper, sliced (80g)
1 medium onion, finely chopped (160g)
2 small celery sticks, finely
   chopped (80g)
1 garlic clove, finely chopped
400g can of chopped tomatoes
1 tsp dried oregano
sea salt and freshly ground black pepper
a little caster sugar, to taste (optional)
50g Parmesan cheese, grated
2 tbsp breadcrumbs (optional)
handful of basil leaves,
   chopped

**5 OF YOUR
5-A-DAY**

Preheat the oven to 200°C/fan 180°C/400°F/gas mark 6.

Mix together half the olive oil with the pesto. Line two baking trays with baking parchment and lay the aubergine and courgette slices on top. Brush one side with the pesto oil. Place the sliced pepper around the slices and roast in the oven for 10 minutes. Turn the slices, brush the other side with the pesto oil and cook the vegetables for another five minutes. Set aside.

Heat the remaining 1 tbsp of oil in a heavy-based saucepan and fry the onion and celery for eight minutes. When soft, add the garlic and cook for a couple of minutes followed by the tomatoes. Add the oregano and allow the tomatoes to reduce for about 30 minutes. When the sauce is thick, add a little salt and sugar (if using) to taste and blitz with a hand-held blender until smooth.

Layer one-third of the tomato sauce in an ovenproof dish, add a good layer of the courgettes and peppers and a sprinkling of Parmesan. Top with another one-third of the sauce, a layer of the aubergines and a bit more Parmesan, finishing with the remaining sauce and any remaining vegetable slices. Mix the remaining Parmesan with the breadcrumbs (if using) and basil and sprinkle on top. Place under the grill or in the hot oven until the top browns.

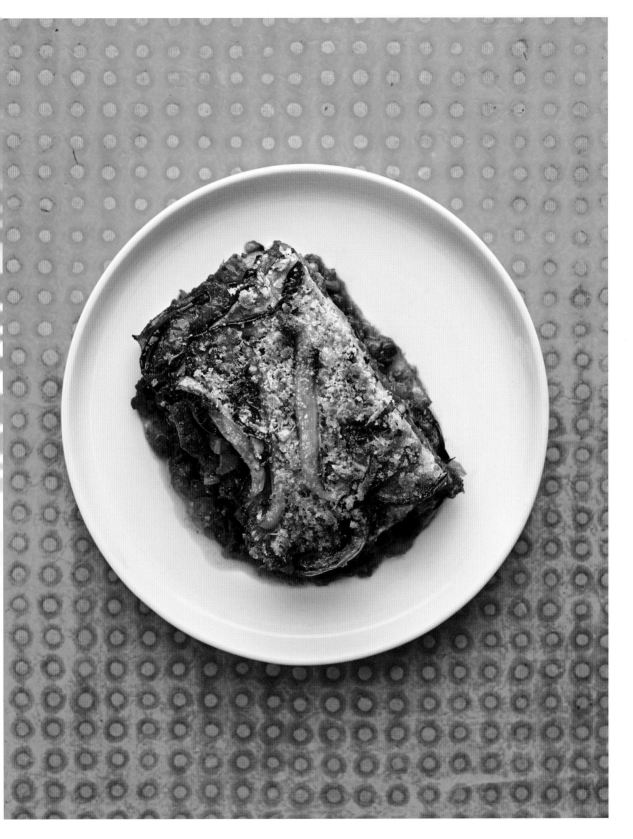

MED VEG AND FETA TART
WITH ONION AND FENNEL JAM | *serves 4 (2 adults; 2 kids)*

This light, savoury tart is based on the French pissaladière and is brimming with vegetables. The sweet smell of puff pastry and roasted vegetables as it comes out of the oven is enough to whet your appetite and the tart looks stunning on the dinner table, too. Great eaten hot or cold.

For the onion and fennel jam

1 tbsp olive oil
2 medium red onions, finely
 sliced (240g)
1 large bulb of fennel, very finely
 sliced (240g)
sea salt and freshly ground black pepper
2 tbsp red wine vinegar
1 tbsp soft brown sugar

For the tart

240g chestnut mushrooms, cut into
 bite-sized pieces
240g cherry tomatoes, halved
1 red pepper, cut into 2cm pieces (160g)
2 tbsp olive oil
a few thyme leaves
120g jarred artichoke hearts, drained
1 tbsp green pesto
375g sheet of ready-rolled puff pastry
1 egg, lightly beaten
100g feta cheese
basil leaves, to serve

**5 OF YOUR
5-A-DAY**

To make the jam, heat the oil in a heavy-based saucepan and add the onions and fennel with ½ tsp salt. Add the vinegar, sugar and about 100ml of water. Bring to the boil, then reduce the heat to a simmer, cover and cook for about one hour until the onions and fennel are reduced, thick and sweet (you may need to add 1 tbsp of water now and again if the onions look like they are drying out too much). Leave to cool.

Meanwhile, for the tart, preheat the oven to 200°C/fan 180°C/400°F/gas mark 6.

Put the mushrooms, tomatoes and pepper in a roasting tin with the oil and a few thyme leaves and place in the oven for about 30 minutes. Once cooked, mix in the artichoke hearts and pesto. Season well with salt and pepper and leave to cool.

Line a baking tray with baking parchment and place the pastry sheet on top. Score the pastry around the edge, leaving a 2.5cm border all round. Prick all over the inner rectangle with a fork and then brush the entire rectangle with the egg. Bake for about 20 minutes until light golden brown (the middle will rise but flatten it before you put the filling on top). This method saves the need for fiddling around with baking beans.

Remove from the oven, flatten the pastry and spread the cooled onion and fennel jam all over the inner rectangle. Top with the roasted vegetables and return to the oven for another 10 minutes until the vegetables are warmed through.

Crumble over the feta and tear over some basil, to serve.

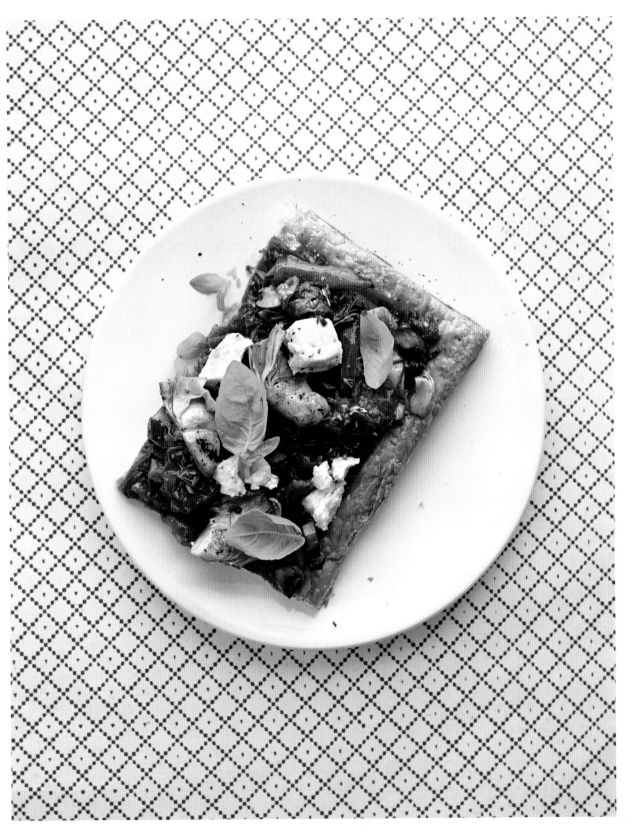

MAGNIFICENT MOUSSAKA | *serves 4 (2 adults; 2 kids)*

A Mediterranean classic made with layered aubergines. This is a really satisfying dish and perfect for a hungry family. Borlotti beans and mushrooms replace the traditional minced lamb, resulting in a meaty taste and texture.

2 large aubergines, sliced into 1cm
  rounds (about 600g)
3 tbsp olive oil, plus more if needed
1 tbsp harissa
2 medium red onions, finely
  chopped (240g)
1 garlic clove, crushed
240g mushrooms, cut into small pieces
400g can of borlotti or pinto beans, with
  the liquid from the can
230g can of chopped tomatoes
1 large ripe tomato, finely
  chopped (80g)
1 tbsp soy sauce
1 tsp Worcestershire sauce
2 tbsp red wine
1 tsp dried oregano
½ tsp dried rosemary
1 bay leaf
sea salt and freshly ground black pepper

For the white sauce
30g unsalted butter
30g plain flour
375ml semi-skimmed milk
100g mature Cheddar cheese, grated
freshly grated nutmeg
1 medium egg, lightly beaten

5 OF YOUR 5-A-DAY

Preheat the oven to 200°C/fan 180°C/400°F/gas mark 6.

Line two baking trays with baking parchment and place the aubergine slices on top. Mix 2 tbsp of the oil with the harissa and brush half the mixture on to one side of the aubergine slices. Bake for five minutes before turning over and brushing the remaining harissa oil on the other side. Cook for a further five minutes, then set aside.

Meanwhile heat the remaining 1 tbsp of oil in a pan and cook the onions over a low heat for about eight minutes until soft. Add the garlic and mushrooms and cook for another five to eight minutes. Add the beans and their liquid together with the canned tomatoes, fresh tomato, soy sauce, Worcestershire sauce, wine, oregano, rosemary and bay leaf. Allow to cook over a medium heat for 20 minutes until reduced and thick. Season with salt and pepper.

For the cheese sauce, put the butter, flour and milk in a saucepan and whisk continuously over a medium heat until the sauce boils and thickens. Reduce the heat and cook for one minute, stirring continuously. Stir in most of the Cheddar, reserving a handful for the top, then add salt, pepper and nutmeg to taste. Leave to cool.

Spread half the bean mixture in an ovenproof dish and cover with half the aubergine slices, season well and top with the rest of the bean mixture. Finish with a final layer of aubergines and season with more salt and pepper.

Mix the egg with the cheese sauce, pour it over the aubergines, sprinkle the remaining cheese on top and bake for about 25 minutes until golden brown.

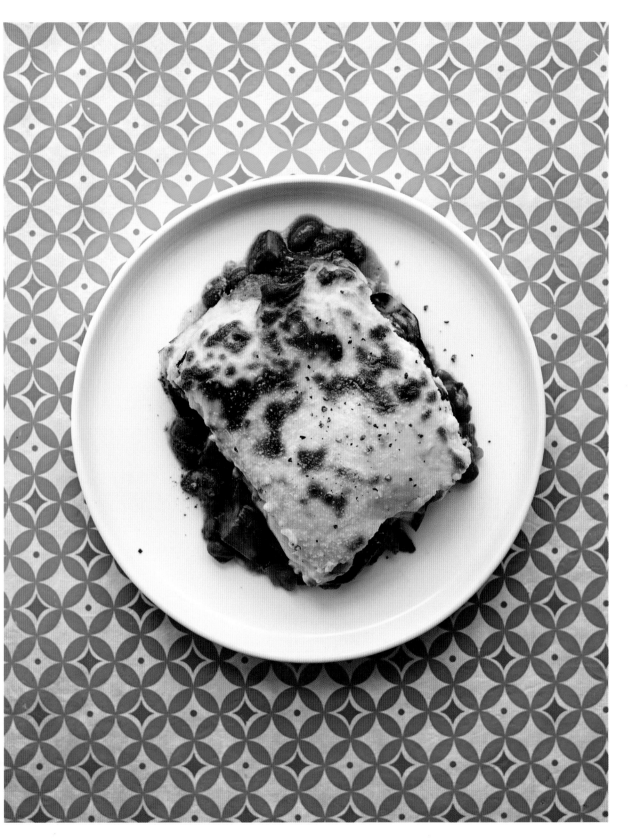

COURGETTE-BASED PIZZA | *serves 4 (2 adults; 2 kids)*

A healthy courgette pizza crust topped with vegetables, this is a great way to encourage your children to eat well as each serving provides five portions of vegetables. It's easy to make, does not need any rising agents and tastes simply scrumptious. Pepperoni can be added, too, if you want.

For the pizza base
1 large courgette (240g)
sea salt
120g strong white flour
80g gram flour
100g mature Cheddar cheese, grated
¼ tsp dried oregano
1 egg, lightly beaten
olive oil, for the tray

For the topping
240g cherry tomatoes, quartered
160g mushrooms, chopped into
  bite-sized pieces
1 garlic clove, finely chopped
handful of basil leaves
1 large red onion, finely sliced (160g)
1 red pepper, finely sliced (160g)
½ yellow pepper, finely sliced (80g)
80g sweetcorn, canned or frozen
50g mature Cheddar cheese, grated

5 OF YOUR 5-A-DAY

Preheat the oven to 240°C/fan 220°C/475°F/gas mark 9.

Start with the pizza base. Leaving the skin on, grate the courgette into a large bowl. Sprinkle with a generous pinch of salt and leave to stand for 15 minutes.

Squeeze the excess moisture out of the courgette and transfer to a large bowl. Add the flours, cheese, ¼ tsp salt, the oregano and finally the egg. Mix until all the ingredients are combined, then use your hands to mix further for a couple of minutes to help activate the gluten in the strong flour. The dough may still be sticky.

Generously oil a non-stick 32cm pizza tray (with holes) and spread the dough on to the tray, then pinch the edges to create a rim. Bake in the oven for 10 minutes. Once cooked, set aside to cool.

Dry-roast the cherry tomatoes and mushrooms for 10 minutes in the oven to release all excess water. Then drain and spread over the base. Sprinkle with the garlic and basil. Spread the onion evenly over the pizza, with the peppers and sweetcorn, followed by the grated cheese. Bake in the oven for a further 18 minutes or until golden brown.

Top Tip: A 40g serving of gram flour counts as one of your five-a-day as it is made from ground chickpeas.

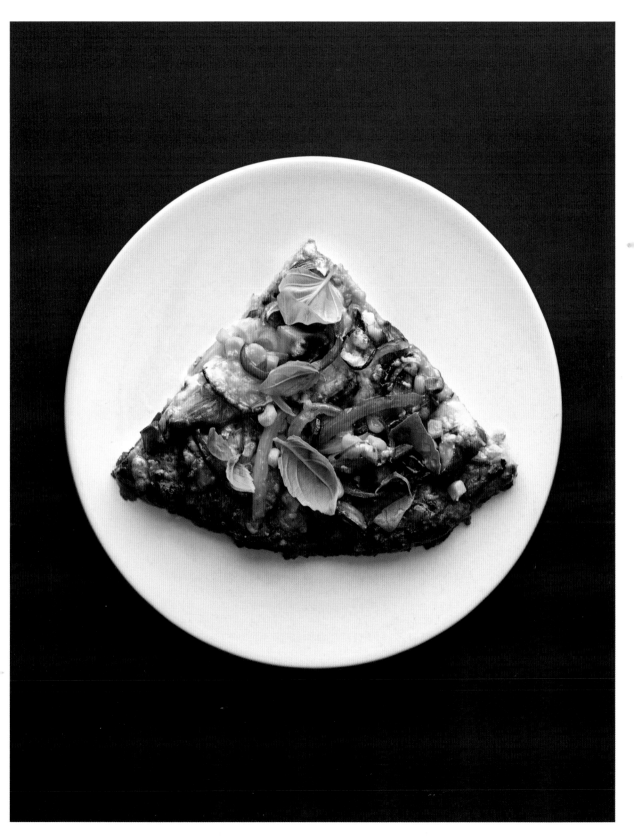

RAINBOW STUFFED PEPPERS | *serves 4 (2 adults; 2 kids)*

This brightly coloured family meal is packed full of tasty vegetables. We use leeks, mushrooms and tomatoes in this version, but any of the kids' favourite vegetables can be used instead. Add couscous for a more substantial meal.

4 peppers (640g)
2 tbsp olive oil
1 large onion, chopped (240g)
3 small leeks, trimmed and
    chopped (240g)
240g chestnut mushrooms, chopped
    into small pieces
sea salt and freshly ground black pepper
3 large tomatoes, chopped (240g)
80g sultanas
80g pine nuts
large handful of chopped mint leaves
3 tbsp balsamic vinegar
100g Parmesan cheese,
    finely grated

5 OF YOUR 5-A-DAY

Put a saucepan of water on to boil. Wash the peppers and slice off the tops. keeping the stalks intact. Remove the seeds and place the peppers (without the tops) in the saucepan of boiling water for two minutes. Drain carefully and run under cold water. Set aside.

Preheat the oven to 200°C/fan 180°C/400°F/gas mark 6.

To prepare the stuffing, heat the oil in a large frying pan and fry the onion, leeks and mushrooms with a little salt for about 10 minutes. When the vegetables are soft and the onion has turned golden, remove from the heat and place in a bowl.

Add the tomatoes, sultanas, pine nuts, mint, balsamic vinegar and half the cheese to the bowl. Mix together and season to taste. Fill the peppers with the stuffing and place in an ovenproof dish, arranging any excess stuffing around the base of the dish. Sprinkle the remaining cheese on top of each filled pepper and replace the pepper 'lids' on the tops.

Bake in the oven for 20 minutes. Eat hot or cold.

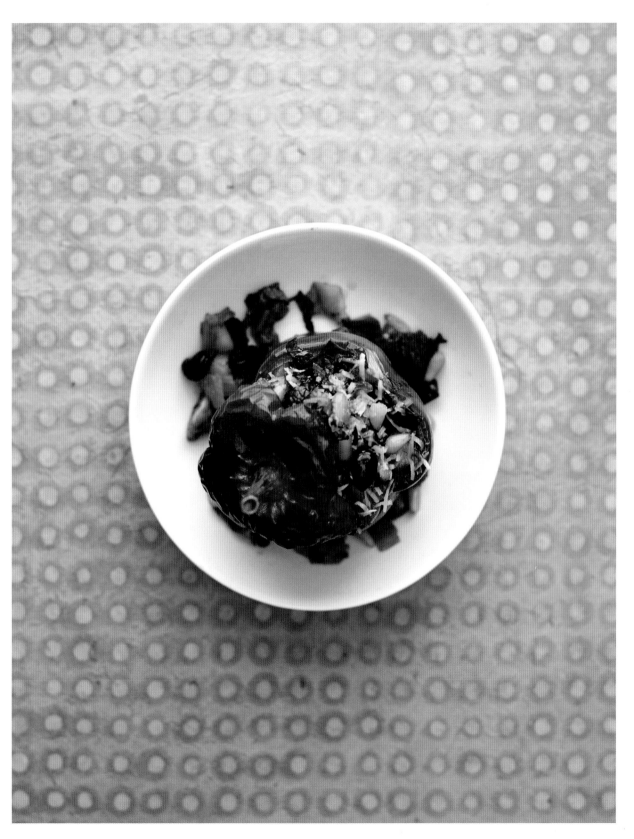

SHEPHERD-LESS PIE | *serves 4 (2 adults; 2 kids)*

A really healthy, nutritious but meat-free alternative to shepherd's pie. The secret to this recipe is the porcini mushrooms, which give a really rich and 'meaty' flavour.

10g dried porcini mushrooms
500g potatoes, peeled
knob of unsalted butter
sea salt and freshly ground black pepper
100g lentilles vertes, or Puy lentils (yields 240g+ when cooked)
2 tbsp sunflower oil
2 medium red onions, chopped (240g)
3 small celery sticks, finely chopped (120g)
1 medium carrot, roughly chopped (120g)
240g chestnut mushrooms, cut into small pieces
¼ x 400g can of chopped tomatoes (about 100g)
2–3 large ripe tomatoes, finely chopped (160g)
1 tsp soy sauce, or to taste
½ tsp Worcestershire sauce, or to taste
40g frozen peas
30g Parmesan cheese, finely grated

5 OF YOUR 5-A-DAY

Soak the porcini in 300ml of warm water for one hour. Retaining the porcini water, strain the mushrooms using a muslin- or kitchen paper-lined sieve. Rinse the porcini to ensure no grit remains.

In the meantime, boil the potatoes for 20 minutes until soft, then drain. Melt the butter in the warm pan and mash the potatoes with the butter and salt and pepper to taste.

Cook the lentils in the porcini water until soft. Once cooked, set aside without draining.

Preheat the oven to 200°C/fan 180°C/400°F/gas mark 6.

Heat the sunflower oil in a heavy-based saucepan and fry the onions for eight minutes until soft. Add the celery and carrot and cook for five to eight minutes before adding the chestnut mushrooms. Cook for five minutes, then add the porcini, the lentils and their cooking water, the canned and fresh tomatoes and the soy sauce and Worcestershire sauce to taste. Cook for 20 minutes, uncovered, until the tomatoes have broken down and lost their acidity. Take off the heat and stir in the peas.

Place in an ovenproof dish and top with the mashed potato. Sprinkle with Parmesan and bake in the oven for 20 minutes until golden brown.

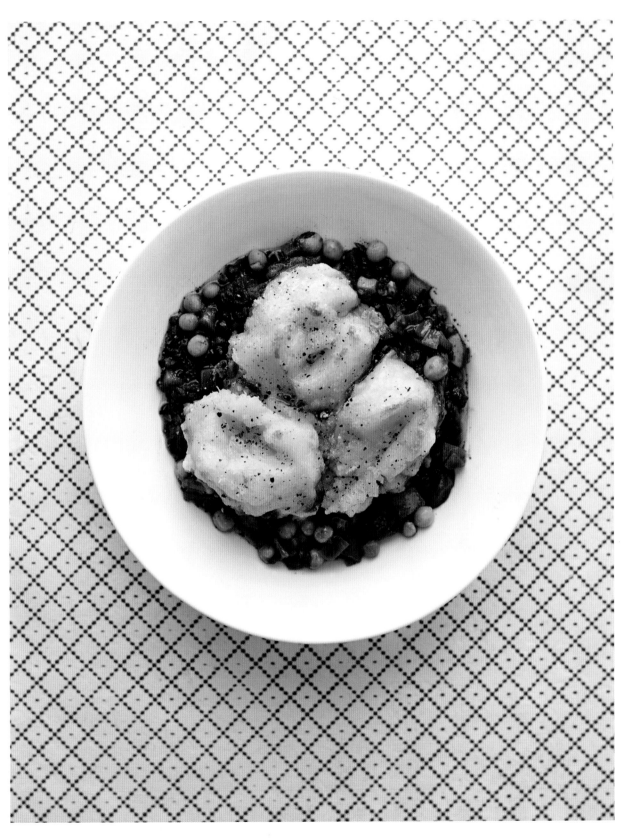

PLIGOURI (BULGAR WHEAT AND VERMICELLI NOODLES) | *serves 2*

Pligouri is traditionally a simple Greek dish of bulgar wheat, which has become a very popular alternative to rice or couscous due to its relatively high nutritional value. Our recipe adds vermicelli for a more interesting texture, with a variety of Mediterranean vegetables.

1 large red onion, chopped into
   bite-sized pieces (160g)
1 courgette, cut into bite-sized
   pieces (160g)
small aubergine, cut into bite-sized
   pieces (160g)
3 tbsp olive oil
2 handfuls of green beans, halved (160g)
2 large handfuls of cherry tomatoes,
   halved (160g)
1 garlic clove, crushed
10 good-quality black olives, pitted
   and halved
2 tsp capers, roughly chopped
3 anchovies, finely chopped (optional)
80g bulgar wheat
80g vermicelli noodles (about 4 nests)
500ml hot chicken or vegetable stock
knob of unsalted butter
large handful of roughly chopped basil
   or parsley leaves
juice of ½ lemon, to serve (optional)
2–3 tbsp Greek yogurt, to serve
   (optional)

5 OF YOUR 5-A-DAY

Preheat the oven to 200°C/fan 180°C/400°F/gas mark 6.

Place the onion, courgette and aubergine in a roasting tin with 2 tbsp of the oil. Roast for about 20 minutes.

Meanwhile, blanch the green beans in salted water for about five minutes, until just done. Drain the beans and return to the warm saucepan with the cherry tomatoes, garlic, olives, capers and anchovies (if using).

Remove the roasting tin from the oven and stir in the green bean mixture. Return to the oven for another 15 minutes.

While that is cooking, heat the remaining 1 tbsp of oil in a pan, add the bulgar wheat and scrunch in each vermicelli nest with your hands to break it up. Ensuring the base of the pan is very hot, add the hot stock (it will bubble vigorously) and immediately cover with a lid. Reduce the heat to its lowest setting and cook for 10 minutes without lifting the lid. After 10 minutes, add the butter to the pan without stirring and remove from the heat. Cover to keep warm.

When the vegetables are cooked, remove from the oven and stir through the basil. Fork through the bulgar mixture and place on a plate topped with the roasted vegetables. Serve with a squeeze of lemon juice and the yogurt, if desired.

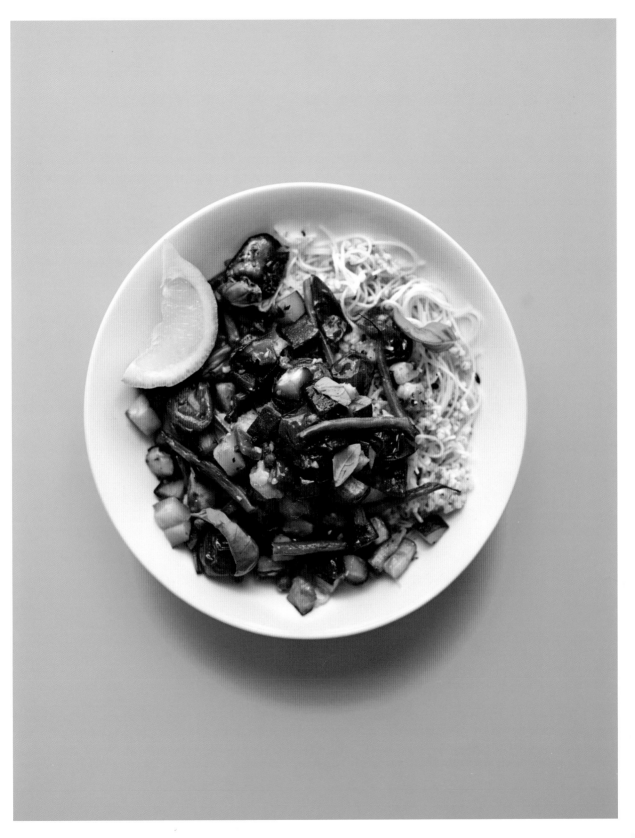

LUSCIOUS LASAGNE | *serves 4 (2 adults; 2 kids)*

Our adapted lasagne recipe uses courgette sheets instead of pasta, making it lighter and lower in carbohydrates. A great family dish, delicious served with hot crusty garlic bread.

3 large courgettes (about 600g)
3 tbsp olive oil
sea salt and freshly ground black pepper
2 medium red onions, finely
 sliced (240g)
1 garlic clove, crushed
240g chestnut mushrooms, cut into
 small bite-sized pieces
small head of broccoli, cut into mini
 florets, stem peeled and grated
 coarsely (240g)
large handful of cherry tomatoes,
 halved (80g)
230g can of chopped tomatoes
2 tsp dried oregano

For the cheese sauce
30g unsalted butter
30g plain flour
375ml semi-skimmed milk
150g Parmesan cheese, finely grated
grated nutmeg, to taste

5 OF YOUR 5-A-DAY

Preheat the oven to 200°C/fan 180°C/400°F/gas mark 6.

Cut each courgette lengthways into about six slices. Brush with olive oil and add freshly ground black pepper. Roast in the oven for 12 minutes, or until lightly coloured.

Put the remaining olive oil in a frying pan and fry the onions for five minutes over a medium heat until lightly coloured. Add the garlic, mushrooms and broccoli florets and fry for a further two to three minutes. Finally, add the fresh and canned tomatoes and dried oregano and cook for 10 minutes until the tomatoes have broken down. Season well.

For the cheese sauce, put the butter, flour and milk in a small saucepan and whisk continuously over a medium heat, until the sauce boils and thickens. Reduce the heat and cook for a further minute, stirring continuously. Remove from the heat, stir in the grated broccoli stems, most of the Parmesan, salt, pepper and nutmeg to taste. Heat for a couple more minutes.

Place half the tomato filling in an ovenproof dish and layer half the courgette slices on top, then half the cheese sauce. Repeat the layering with the other half of the filling, then the remaining courgette slices and finally the last of the cheese sauce. Sprinkle over the remaining Parmesan and place in the oven for 20 minutes until golden brown.

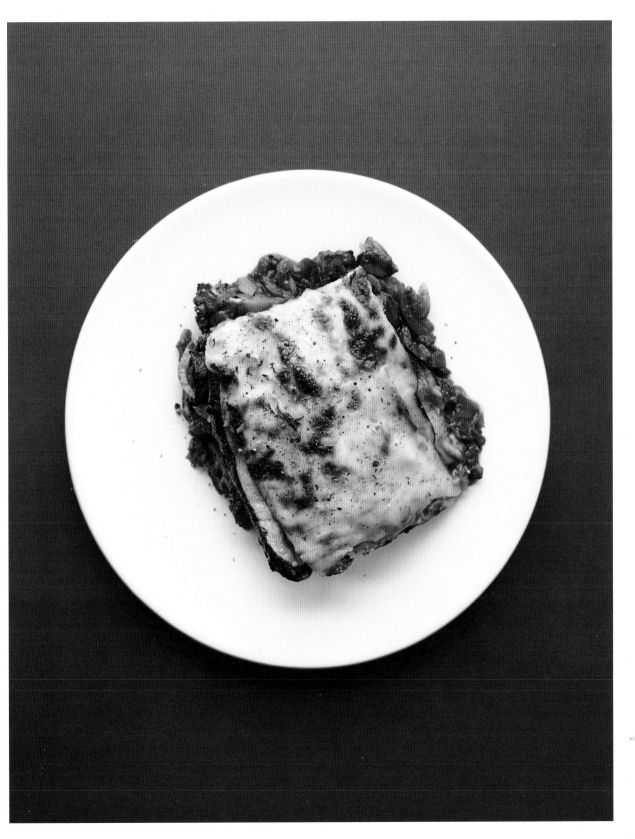

CHEESY MAC 'N' VEG | *serves 2 kids*
(5 x 40g portions of veg each)

Pasta and cheese is a universal favourite amongst kids, so it's a wise choice for sneaking in a few extra veg. Our cheese sauce recipe is really quick and easy, although a shop-bought version would make this dish super-convenient (but home-made tastes better!). This is delicious with bacon, too.

For the cheese sauce
EITHER
25g unsalted butter
25g plain flour
300ml milk
pinch of freshly grated nutmeg
75g mature Cheddar cheese, grated,
  plus more for the top
sea salt and freshly ground black pepper
OR
350g tub of ready-made cheese sauce

For the rest
100g macaroni or penne
1 tbsp unsalted butter
1 small leek, trimmed and finely
  sliced (80g)
handful of cauliflower florets, broken
  into small pieces (80g)
handful of broccoli florets, broken into
  small pieces (80g)
3 heaped tbsp frozen peas,
  defrosted (80g)
80g spinach, shredded

**5 OF YOUR
5-A-DAY**

Preheat the oven to 200°C/fan 180°C/400°F/gas mark 6.

Make the cheese sauce (if making home-made) by putting all the ingredients except the cheese in a small saucepan. Whisk continuously over a medium heat until the sauce boils and thickens. Reduce the heat and cook for a further minute, stirring continuously. Remove from the heat, stir in the cheese and season to taste.

Boil some water with a pinch of salt and cook the pasta according to the packet instructions.

Meanwhile, heat the 1 tbsp of butter in a heavy-based saucepan and sauté the leek for a couple of minutes, then add the cauliflower and broccoli. Continue cooking for about five minutes until the cauliflower and broccoli have softened. Add the peas and spinach and cook for a further two minutes until the spinach has wilted.

Mix the vegetables with 1 tbsp of the cheese sauce and spoon into an ovenproof dish. Mix the pasta with the remaining cheese sauce and lay on top of the vegetables. Sprinkle with some grated cheese and bake for about 20 minutes until golden brown on top.

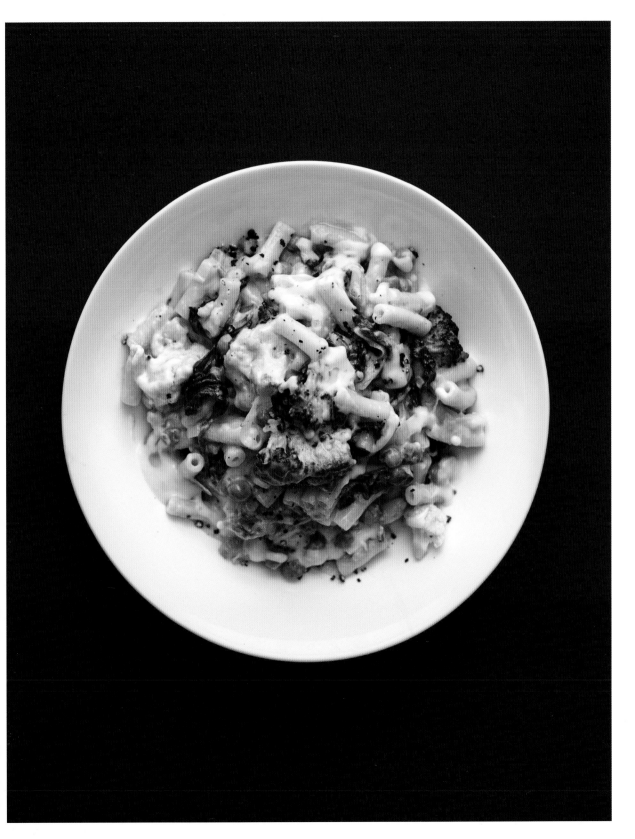

CALZONE BITES | *serves 2 kids*
(5 x 40g portions of veg each)

These are super-moreish and quick to make. A firm favourite with the kids, they provide a generous and healthy snack and are very popular with adults, too! Adding a handful of chopped ham or pepperoni will satisfy the carnivores in your family.

1 small red onion, finely chopped (80g)
½ red pepper, finely chopped (80g)
80g mushrooms, finely sliced
1 tbsp olive oil
80g canned or frozen sweetcorn
80g spinach, shredded
sea salt and freshly ground black pepper
2 large flour tortillas
2 tbsp ready-made pizza sauce, or
  Tomato sauce (see page 130)
80g Cheddar cheese,
  finely grated

**5 OF YOUR
5-A-DAY**

Fry the onion, red pepper and mushrooms in the oil for about 10 minutes until softened and reduced in volume. Stir in the sweetcorn and spinach and cook until the spinach has wilted. Season with salt and pepper.

Spread one tortilla with 1 tbsp of the pizza sauce, making sure it goes to the edges. Place in a dry, large non-stick frying pan over a medium heat. Sprinkle one-quarter of the cheese over half the tortilla and lay half the filling on top. Sprinkle another one-quarter of the cheese on top and fold the tortilla over to create a semi-circle. Fry on each side for two or three minutes until golden and the cheese has started to melt.

Remove from the pan and allow to cool a little while you cook the other tortilla. With a serrated knife, carefully cut each semi-circle into three triangles and serve.

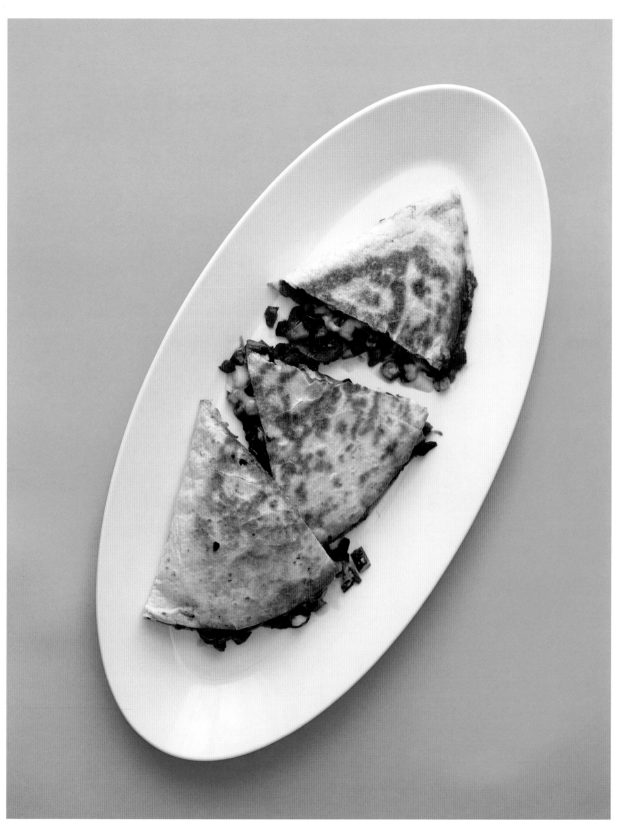

QUICK EGG-FRIED RICE | *serves 2 kids*
(5 x 40g portions of veg each)

Most kids love egg-fried rice, so combining it with their favourite vegetables makes for a quick and easy supper. This recipe uses ginger and garlic but, if they are not to the kids' taste, simply leave them out and finish with some cheese instead (but leave out the soy sauce if you're using cheese). This is good with chicken, too.

1 tbsp oil
1 small red onion, finely chopped (80g)
½ red pepper, finely chopped (80g)
handful of broccoli florets, broken into
   very small pieces (about 80g)
2 tsp finely chopped root ginger
   (optional)
1 garlic clove, finely chopped (optional)
2 eggs, lightly beaten
250g cold cooked rice
handful of baby sweetcorn, or 3 tbsp
   canned sweetcorn (80g)
3 heaped tbsp frozen peas,
   defrosted (80g)
2 tsp light soy sauce

**5 OF YOUR
5-A-DAY**

Heat half the oil in a wok and fry the onion, pepper, broccoli, ginger and garlic. Stir-fry for three minutes, then break in the eggs, stirring them around to scramble.

Once the eggs have cooked, remove the mixture from the pan. Clean the wok and heat the remaining oil. Stir-fry the cooked rice for five minutes until piping hot, then add the cooked vegetables with the sweetcorn and peas and heat until hot through.

Add the soy sauce and serve.

Top Tip Be careful when using cold cooked rice that you cool the rice quickly and cover and refrigerate it as soon as possible; use within two days.

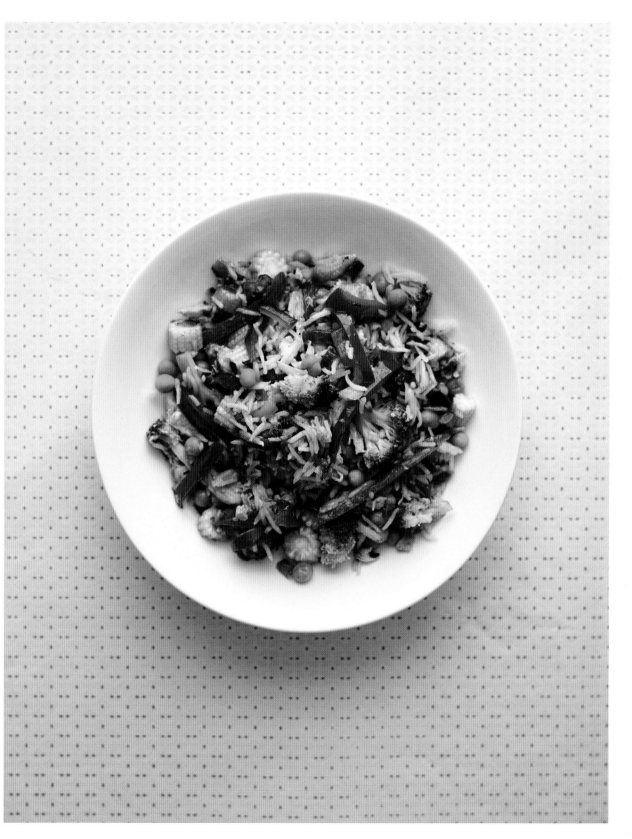

MEAN BALLS WITH TOMATO SAUCE

serves 4 kids (5 x 40g portions of veg each)

These spicy veggie mean balls look just like traditional meat balls and taste just as good, too. Served with a wholesome tomato sauce, this is a perfect way to give the kids their five-a-day.

For the mean balls

1 tbsp sunflower oil, plus more to fry
small red onion, finely chopped (80g)
1 small carrot, coarsely grated (80g)
80g mushrooms, finely chopped
400g can of borlotti beans, drained and
   rinsed (net weight 240g)
1 garlic clove, finely chopped
1 tsp ground cumin
1 tsp ground coriander
½ tsp mustard
1 tsp soy sauce
1 tsp finely chopped rosemary
4 tbsp oats

For the tomato sauce

1 tbsp sunflower oil
1 small onion, finely chopped (80g)
1 small courgette, finely chopped (80g)
½ red pepper, finely chopped (80g)
1 garlic clove, finely chopped
400g can of chopped tomatoes
sea salt and freshly ground
   black pepper

5 OF YOUR 5-A-DAY

Heat the oil in a frying pan and sauté the onion, carrot and mushrooms for about 10 minutes until soft.

Meanwhile, pat the drained borlotti beans dry with kitchen paper. Put the beans and everything else for the mean balls into a food processor (not the contents of the frying pan just yet, though) and pulse-blend until you have a coarse mixture. Empty into a bowl and stir through the cooked onion, carrot and mushroom mixture. Form into 12–16 balls and place in the fridge for 20 minutes.

Meanwhile, make the tomato sauce: heat the oil in a pan and add the onion, courgette, pepper and garlic. Cook for seven to 10 minutes until softened. Add the tomatoes with 100ml of water and a pinch of salt and pepper. Cook over a medium heat for 30 minutes, adding extra water only if necessary. Leave to cool for a few minutes, then blend until smooth.

Heat some oil in a non-stick frying pan, add the mean balls and fry for eight minutes over a medium heat, turning halfway through. Serve with the tomato sauce and some pasta.

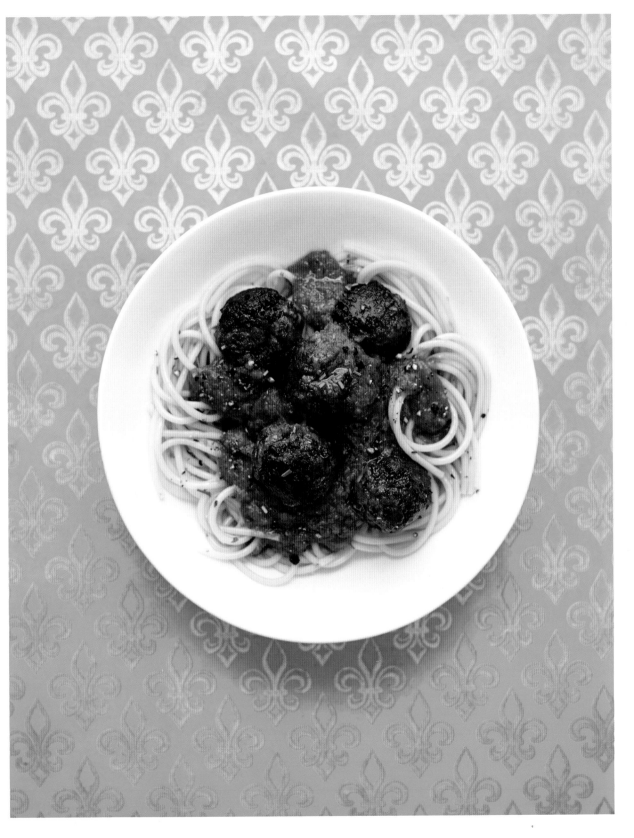

SPRING ROCK 'N' ROLLS | *serves 4 kids (makes 8)*
(5 x 40g portions of veg each)

These crispy, golden spring rolls are certain to tempt your kids into eating more vegetables. The cabbage and beansprouts almost act as a substitute for noodles and the kids devour them without even noticing what's inside! You can add any finely sliced vegetables, or even cooked chicken, to the recipe.

1 tbsp oil, plus more to deep-fry
1 tbsp finely chopped root ginger
1 garlic clove, finely chopped
4 banana shallots, finely sliced (160g)
1 medium carrot, grated (80g)
handful of mange tout, shredded (80g)
160g mushrooms, finely sliced
½ head of Chinese leaf,
   shredded (160g)
160g beansprouts
1 tbsp soy sauce
1 tsp tomato ketchup (optional; it makes
   the filling sweeter)
8 sheets of filo pastry
a little plain flour

**5 OF YOUR
5-A-DAY**

Heat the oil in a wok and stir-fry the ginger, garlic and shallots for two minutes. Add the carrot, mange tout, mushrooms, cabbage and beansprouts and continue stir-frying for about eight minutes until soft and reduced in volume. Add the soy sauce and ketchup (if using).

To make the spring rolls, take one sheet of filo pastry and fold in half so you have a rectangle in front of you. Place one-eighth of the mixture about 2.5cm from the edge nearest you, carefully fold in the sides and roll up the spring roll. In a small bowl, mix the flour with water to make a paste and use this to seal the spring roll shut. Repeat to make eight rolls.

Heat the oil for deep-frying in a small saucepan to 180°C/350°F, using a cook's thermometer. Be careful to keep an eye on it. When the required temperature is reached, carefully lower a couple of the spring rolls into the oil. Cook for two or three minutes, turning regularly with a metal spoon, until golden brown.

Remove, drain on kitchen paper and keep warm while you cook the remaining spring rolls.

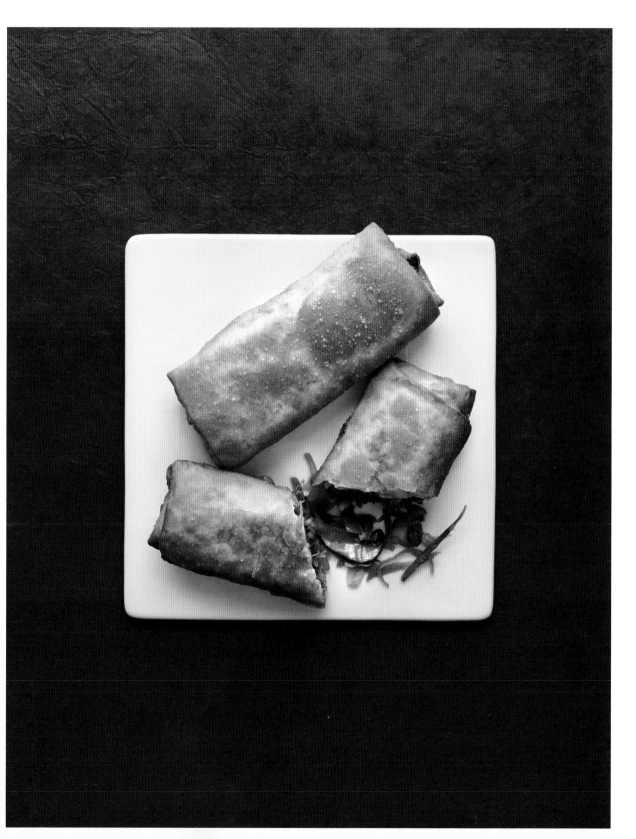

TOP UP YOUR 5: SNACKS

Up to this point, all the recipes in this book have contained all five portions of your five-a-day. But we realise it's not always possible to get your quota in this way. In this chapter we give recipes which include anything from one to four portions, adapting snacking favourites to include a few more vegetables. So whether you are looking for something to eat on the go, grazing in front of the TV, or preparing pre-dinner nibbles, there's something here to help you sneak in more veg.

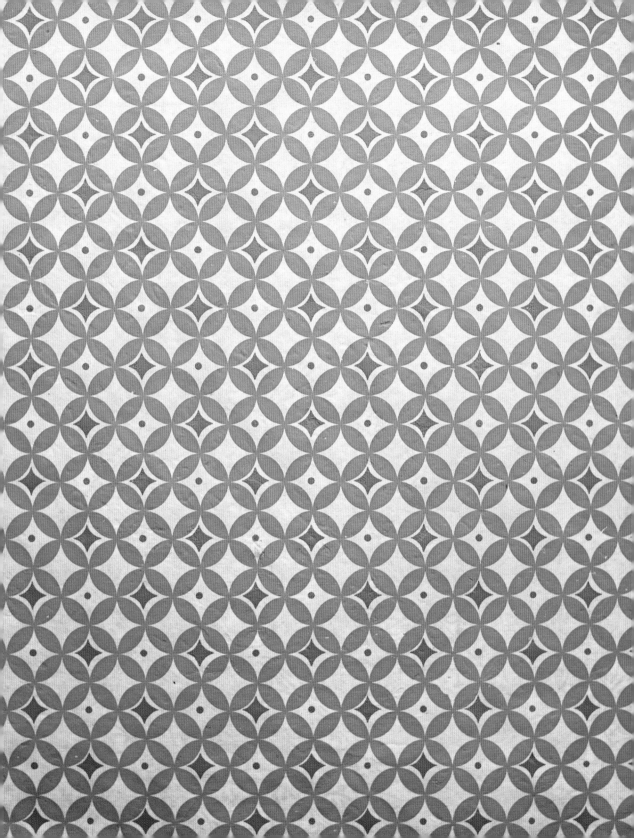

VEGETABLE AND HOUMOUS WRAP | *serves 2*

These are delicious and are a really convenient way to up your five-a-day on the go. They're perfect for the kids to snack on, too. Make enough houmous for the week ahead; that way there's always something healthy at hand.

1 red pepper, sliced (160g)
½ yellow pepper, sliced (80g)
1 small red onion, cut into bite-sized
   pieces (80g)
a little olive oil
2 heaped tbsp Houmous
   (see page 152)
2 large seeded wraps
1 large avocado, sliced (160g)
5cm piece of cucumber, sliced (80g)

4 OF YOUR 5-A-DAY

Preheat the oven to 200°C/fan 180°C/400°F/gas mark 6. Toss the peppers and red onion in the oil and roast for about 25 minutes, or until soft.

To assemble the wraps, spread half the houmous over each wrap. Place half the roasted vegetables, avocado and cucumber in the middle of each. Roll up the wraps, tucking in the sides as you go. Cut at an angle and serve.

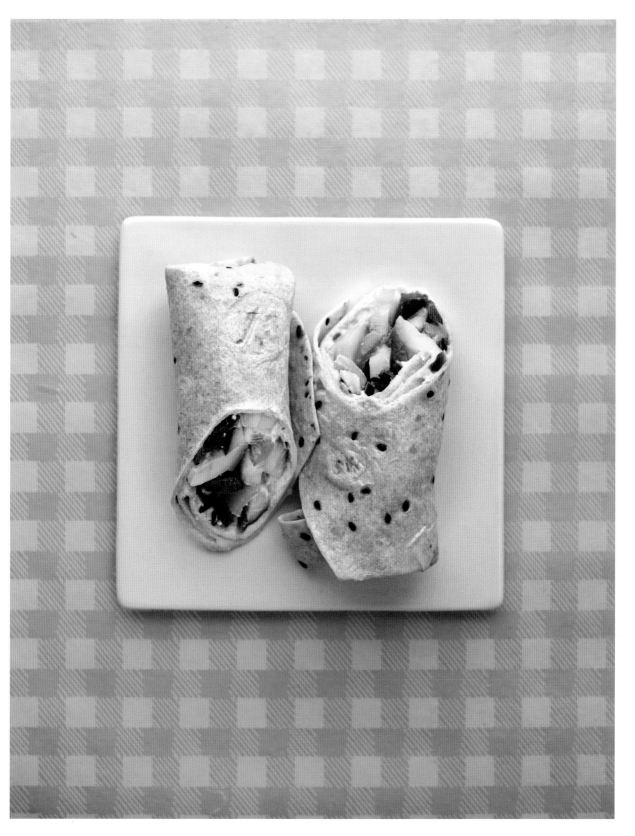

SWEET POTATO AND COURGETTE FALAFEL | *serves 8 (makes 32)*

This snack is traditionally deep-fried, but our healthier falafel are baked. We also use sweet potato and courgette to give a really light and nutritious snack. The trick here is to use raw chickpeas (soaked overnight), as using canned will make the mixture too wet. This recipe makes quite a lot, but the falafel freeze very well, so are ultra-handy to have in stock.

400g sweet potato, peeled and cut
  into chunks
200g dried chickpeas, soaked for
  24 hours, then drained
1 large courgette, chopped (200g)
1 large onion, chopped (200g)
3–5 garlic cloves, crushed
3 large handfuls of herbs (any mixture of
  coriander, mint and parsley leaves)
1 tbsp ground cumin
sea salt and freshly ground black pepper
4 tbsp sunflower oil,
  plus more to bake

2 OF YOUR 5-A-DAY

Boil the sweet potato until tender, then drain well and mash.

Combine the remaining ingredients – except the oil to bake – in a food processor and blitz until a coarse texture is formed. Stir in the sweet potato by hand. If the mixture feels too wet to form into balls, drain a little of the liquid: you can do this by placing the mixture in a sieve over a bowl and pressing down, or by placing some in a tea towel and squeezing it out. For best results, then spread the mixture out on a baking tray and leave in the fridge for a few hours to dry out a little more.

Make into small balls, each the size of a large cherry tomato and flatten slightly. Open-freeze on a baking sheet, separated by layers of greaseproof paper. When frozen solid, tip into a large freezer bag.

When required, preheat the oven to 200°C/fan 180°C/ 400°F/gas mark 6. Brush the falafel with a little oil and bake for 30 minutes, turning halfway through.

Top Tip: Make these in big batches and freeze them as the best results are achieved by baking straight from frozen, which makes them a hugely convenient standby.

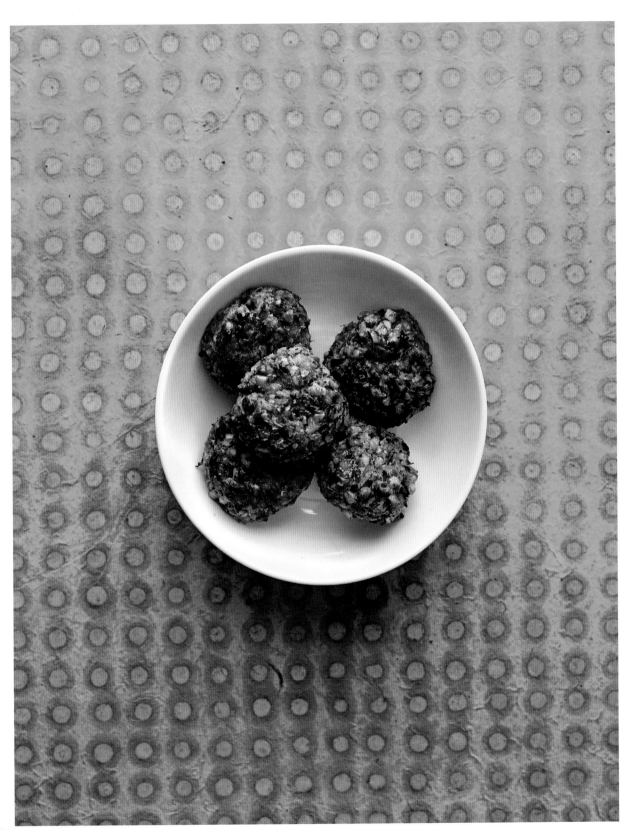

COURGETTE, CARROT AND FETA FRITTERS | *serves 2 (makes 6)*

These are most delicious hot and fresh out of the pan, but nearly as tasty cold. They are also healthier than deep-fried versions. An ideal on-the-go snack or for kids' packed lunches.

1 courgette (160g)
1 small carrot (80g)
1 small onion, very finely sliced (80g)
1 egg, lightly beaten
2 tbsp plain flour
1 tsp baking powder
50g feta cheese, crumbled
handful of mint leaves
1 tsp finely grated unwaxed lemon zest
   (optional)
sea salt and freshly ground black pepper
2 tbsp sunflower oil

2 OF YOUR 5-A-DAY

Using the coarse side of a grater, grate the courgette and carrot. Mix with the onion in a bowl together with the egg, flour, baking powder, feta, mint and lemon zest. Season with a little salt and plenty of pepper.

Heat the sunflower oil in a frying pan. Using half the mixture, make three fritters in the pan, each about the size of your palm. Fry for at least five minutes over a medium-high heat, allowing a deep golden crust to form before carefully turning. Fry on the other side over a slightly lower heat for a further five to seven minutes, or until cooked. Keep warm while you repeat with the other half of the mixture to make a further three fritters.

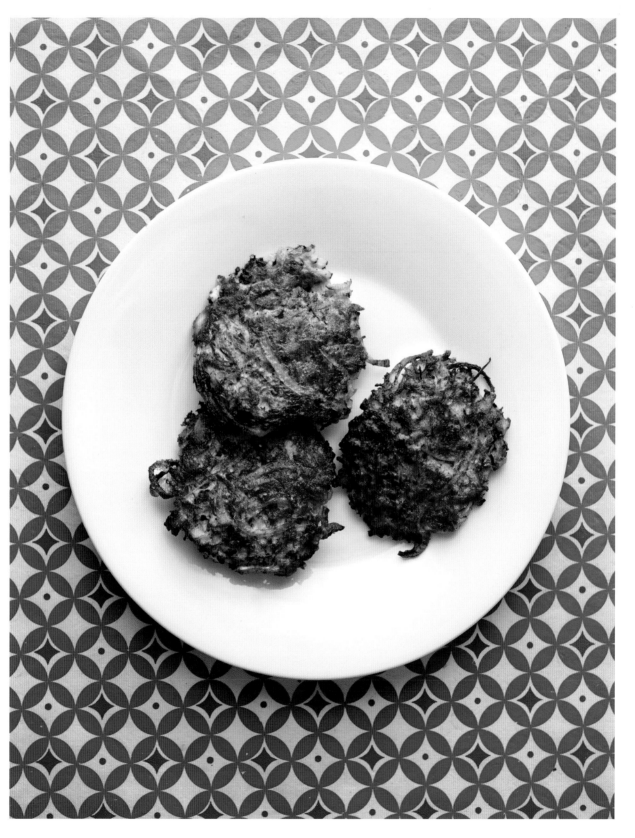

ONION AND PARSNIP
BHAJIS | *serves 2 (makes 6–8)*

A vegetable fritter from India, these bhajis make a delicious appetiser, light snack or accompaniment to a curry. Perfect with Cucumber and banana raita (see page 170).

80g gram flour
40g rice flour
juice of ½ lemon
1 tsp cumin seeds
½ tsp ground turmeric
¼ tsp chilli powder
1 garlic clove, finely chopped
1 tsp grated root ginger
2 tbsp chopped coriander leaves
sea salt
1 small red onion, thinly sliced (80g)
1 small parsnip, cut into thin strips (80g)
sunflower oil, to deep-fry

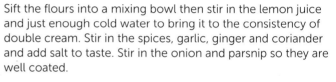

2 OF YOUR 5-A-DAY

Sift the flours into a mixing bowl then stir in the lemon juice and just enough cold water to bring it to the consistency of double cream. Stir in the spices, garlic, ginger and coriander and add salt to taste. Stir in the onion and parsnip so they are well coated.

Heat the oil in a deep-fat fryer to 180°C/350°F on an oil thermometer. Once the oil is up to temperature, make tablespoon-sized bhajis and drop into the hot oil (do not crowd the pan; cook in batches if necessary). Stir carefully to stop them sticking to each other. Cook for about three minutes, turning occasionally, until golden.

Drain on kitchen paper and keep warm while you fry the rest.

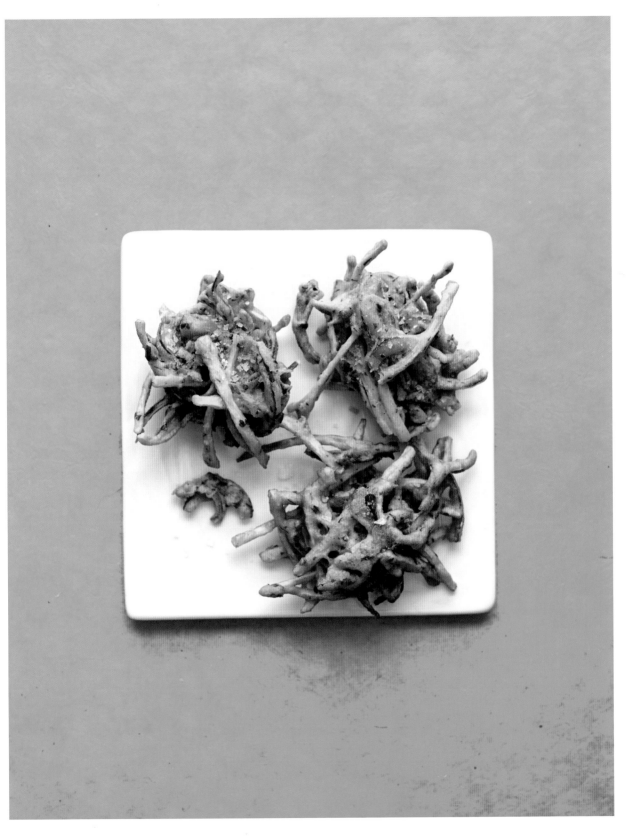

THRIVE ON FIVE'S FAMOUS PASTY | *serves 2*

This is one of our earliest and most popular creations. Delicious puff pastry encases a succulent filling that is meat-free but maintains that peppery pasty bite.

1 tbsp oil
1 medium onion, finely chopped (160g)
160g swede, coarsely grated
160g mushrooms, roughly chopped
sea salt and freshly ground black pepper
40g Cheddar cheese, grated
1 tsp wholegrain mustard
375g sheet of ready-rolled puff pastry
1 egg, lightly beaten

3 OF YOUR 5-A-DAY

Heat the oil in a heavy-based saucepan and fry the onion, swede and mushrooms with a little salt for about 20 minutes until all the vegetables are soft and reduced in volume

When the mixture has cooled a bit, add the cheese, mustard and plenty of black pepper.

Preheat the oven to 200°C/fan 180°C/400°F/gas mark 6.

Cover a baking tray with baking parchment. Cut out two 20cm discs of pastry using a side plate as a guide and place them on the baking parchment.

Place half the filling in the middle of each pastry, brush one edge with egg and gather up both edges to seal. Crimp and fold to form two pasties. Make one small slit in the tops to allow steam to escape, brush with the egg and bake in the oven for about 25 minutes until golden brown. (There will be more pastry than you need; freeze it for another time.)

Leave to cool on a wire rack for a few minutes before serving.

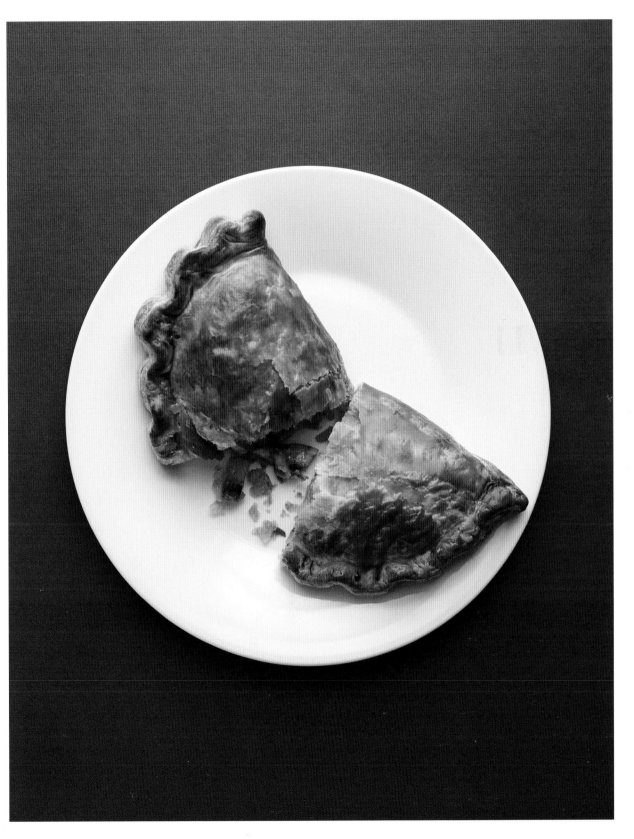

ROAST MED VEG WRAP | *serves 2*

To ensure you get a really healthy wrap, it's best to put it together yourself. Due to their shape, you can squeeze in plenty of vegetables. These wraps are ideal to eat on-the-go and are also perfect for the packed lunch box.

1 medium onion, sliced into thickish
  rounds (160g)
1 Romano pepper, cut into large
  chunks (120g)
½ aubergine, cut into half moons (160g)
1 tbsp olive oil
sea salt and freshly ground black pepper
60g sun-blushed tomatoes or Slow-
  roasted tomatoes (see page 32)
40g olives, pitted and chopped
2 large seeded wraps

**4 OF YOUR
5-A-DAY**

Preheat the oven to 200°C/fan 180°C/400°F/gas mark 6.

Place the onion, pepper and aubergine in a roasting tin with the oil and cook for 30 minutes. Once cooked, season well, add the sun-blushed tomatoes and olives and mix.

Take 1 tbsp of the mix and mash a little with a fork. Spread this over a wrap before adding half of the unmashed mix in the middle. Fold up the wrap, tucking in the sides. Repeat to roll the second wrap. Cut each in half with a serrated knife.

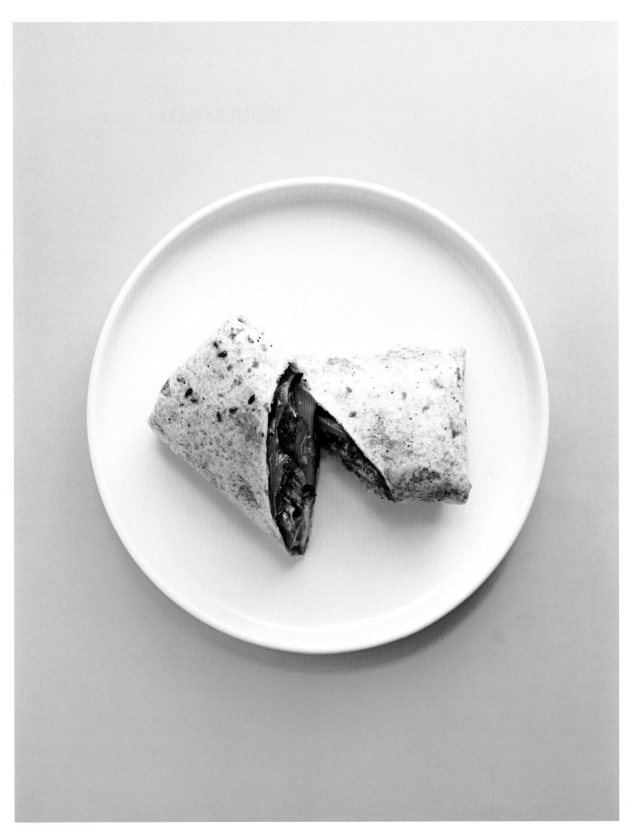

COURGETTE FRITTATA | *serves 4*

*A golden frittata, delicious eaten hot or cold. Perfect as a
snack to top up your five-a-day, or served with a salad as
a light main course.*

3 tbsp olive oil
2 medium onions, finely sliced (320g)
sea salt and freshly ground black pepper
2 courgettes, sliced 5mm thick (320g)
35g Parmesan cheese, grated
2 medium eggs, lightly beaten

2 OF YOUR
5-A-DAY

Heat 1 tbsp of the oil in a large frying pan and fry the onions
with a pinch of salt for about eight minutes. When the onions
are soft and sweet, remove from the pan and set aside.

In the same pan, heat another 1 tbsp of oil and fry the
courgette slices until lightly golden on both sides (about
10 minutes).

Place the onions and courgettes in a bowl and stir in the
Parmesan and eggs. Season with salt and pepper. Preheat the
grill to its highest setting.

The frittata should be quite small and thick, like a cake, so
take a small (15cm) frying pan, heat the remaining 1 tbsp of
oil and fry the mixture over a medium heat for three to four
minutes. Place the pan under the hot grill until the top sets
and is lightly golden. Making sure you protect your hands with
oven gloves or a tea towel, flip the frittata out of the pan on
to a board to serve.

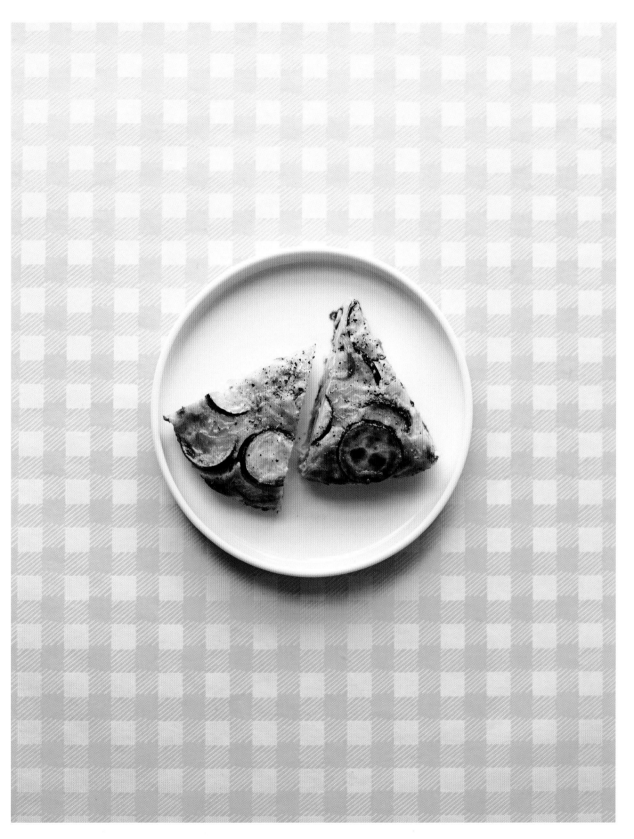

CORN, SPINACH AND CHILLI EMPANADAS | *serves 4 (makes 8)*

A South American version of the Cornish pasty, our empanada recipe uses ready-made pastry, meaning these are quick to make. No need to pre-cook anything, just mix and pop in the oven for a really tasty snack.

240g spinach
60g canned sweetcorn
2 spring onions (20g)
½ red chilli
30g mature Cheddar cheese, grated
½ tsp mustard
a little chopped coriander (optional)
sea salt and freshly ground black pepper
400g sheet of ready-rolled
   shortcrust pastry
1 egg, lightly beaten

1 OF YOUR 5-A-DAY

Preheat the oven to 200°C/fan 180°C/400°F/gas mark 6.

Put the spinach in a colander, pour over boiling water to wilt completely, squeeze out the excess water and chop. In a bowl, mix the spinach, sweetcorn, spring onions, chilli, cheese, mustard, coriander, salt and plenty of pepper.

Cut the pastry into eight even-sized discs using a 12.5cm circle as a guide (probably a large mug or small saucer; check your cupboards). Divide the mixture between them. Gently fold the pastry over to form a semi-circle and seal the edge with a little egg before crimping with a fork or your fingers. Brush the empanadas with more egg and place on a tray lined with greaseproof paper.

Bake for about 25 minutes. Leave to cool for a few minutes, then serve.

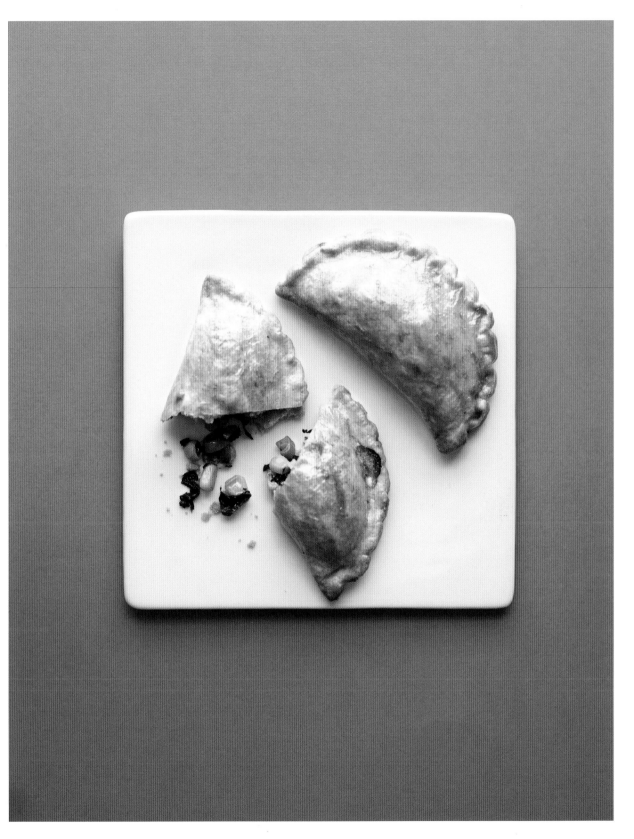

HOUMOUS WITH CLUTCH BAG CRUDITES | *serves 2*

Don't worry, we are not trying to tell you that crudités are a recipe! Let's face it though: eating raw veg is the simplest way of getting five-a-day. But they can be a tough sell. So we pair them here with one of the simplest and most appealing dips to make and eat. Getting into the crudité habit will serve you well... Put a few in your bag to take to work, or into a lunch box and serve them with the houmous, or with any of our delicious dips (see pages 164–181).

For the houmous
400g can of chickpeas (net weight 240g), drained, but reserve some liquid from the can
1 tbsp tahini
2 garlic cloves, crushed
1 tsp finely grated unwaxed lemon zest (optional)
1 tbsp olive oil
sprinkling of ground cumin
sea salt and freshly ground black pepper

For the crudités
1 large carrot, cut into sticks (160g)
½ cucumber, cut into sticks (160g)
1 red pepper, sliced (160g)
4 small celery sticks (160g)
2 handfuls of radishes or a 20cm piece of mooli (160g)

Make the houmous by putting everything in a food processor, including 2 tbsp of the reserved chickpea liquid, and process until smooth. Add more chickpea liquid until you get the desired consistency and season with salt and pepper.

Serve with the crudités.

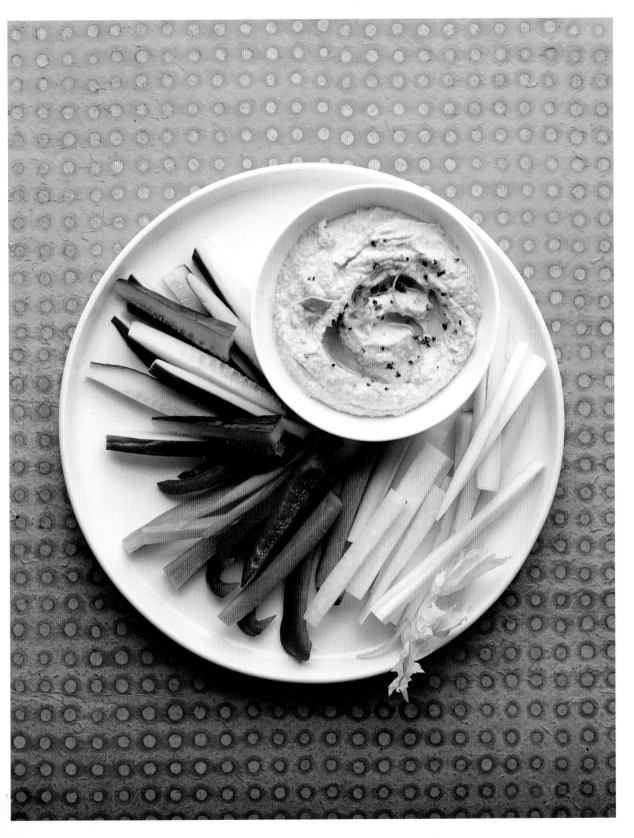

HERBY STUFFED MUSHROOMS | *serves 4 (makes 8)*

Great as a light lunch or as a starter, these stuffed mushrooms look so enticing straight out of the oven and are full of flavour. The 'stuffing' can be made up to two days in advance, making these very easy to assemble when you are ready to serve.

2 tbsp sunflower oil
8 medium portobellini mushrooms, centre stems removed (320g in total)
2 small leeks, trimmed and finely sliced (160g)
2 large fresh tomatoes, finely chopped (160g)
2 tbsp pine nuts
2 tsp chopped sage or tarragon leaves
30g Parmesan cheese, finely grated
sea salt and freshly ground black pepper

2 OF YOUR 5-A-DAY

Preheat the oven to 220°C/fan 200°C/425°F/gas mark 7.

Heat 1 tbsp of oil in a large frying pan, place over a medium-high heat and fry the mushrooms on each side for one minute. Set aside.

In the same pan, add the remaining oil and gently fry the leeks for about 10 minutes until soft and sweet. Put into a bowl with the tomatoes and pine nuts. Add the herbs and half the cheese and mix well. Season to taste.

Place the mushrooms in a shallow ovenproof dish and top each one with the leek and tomato mixture. Sprinkle over the remaining Parmesan and cook in the oven for 15–20 minutes until golden on top.

Leave to cool for five minutes before serving warm.

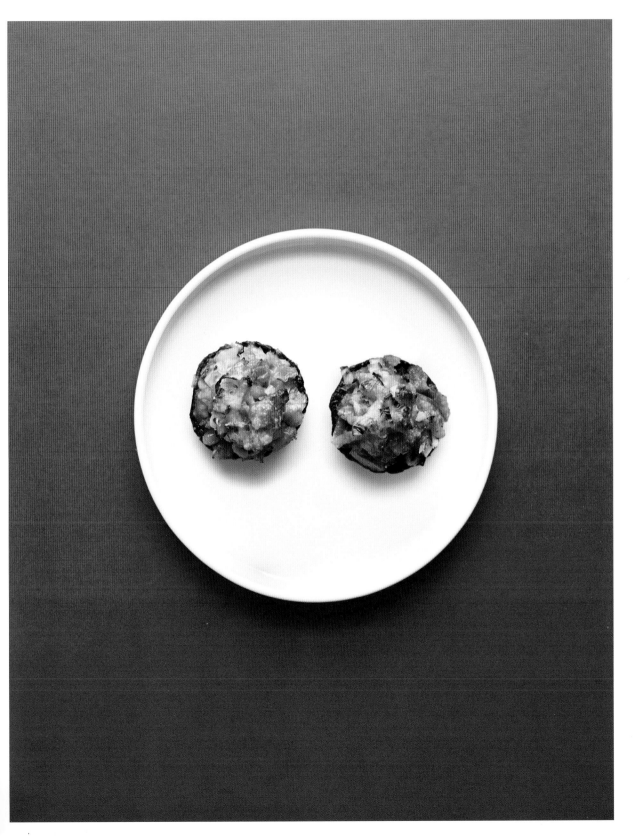

VEGETABLE TEMPURA

serves 2 (enough batter for 5 portions of veg each)

If you're ever struggling to get anyone to eat more vegetables, dipping them in batter is bound to do the trick! These light and crispy tempura are a perfect appetiser or snack. You can use almost any type of vegetable; this is a great way to make sure leftovers are used up at the end of the week.

For the dipping sauce (optional)
3 tbsp Japanese soy sauce
1 tbsp mirin

For the vegetables (80g of any of the following count as one portion) choose from: *asparagus, aubergine, baby sweetcorn, broccoli florets, carrot, cauliflower florets, Chinese leaf, courgette, mushroom, parsnip, spring onions*

For the batter and to fry
flavourless vegetable oil, to deep-fry
100g plain flour, plus more to coat
40g cornflour
½ tsp baking powder
½ tsp salt
200–225ml very cold sparkling water
2 ice cubes

UP TO 5
OF YOUR
5-A-DAY

First make the dipping sauce (if using) by mixing the ingredients. Set aside.

Slice the vegetables into 5mm slices, or chunks, as appropriate to their shape.

Heat the oil for deep-frying in a small saucepan to 180°C/350°F, using a cook's thermometer. Be careful to keep an eye on it while making the batter.

You need to make the batter immediately before you intend to fry. Place the flours, baking powder and salt in a bowl. Slowly add the water, mixing lightly with a pair of chopsticks, until you have the consistency of single cream. It's important not to over-mix as you don't want to activate the gluten (and don't worry about any lumps that remain). Add a couple of ice cubes to the batter and sit the mixture over a bowl of iced water (it's important that the batter remains cold).

When you are ready to fry, place a couple of tablespoons of plain flour in a bowl and use this to coat the vegetables lightly before dipping in the batter (it helps the batter to stick). Fry in the hot oil until lightly golden.

Drain on kitchen paper while you quickly cook the remaining vegetables. Serve with the dipping sauce (if using).

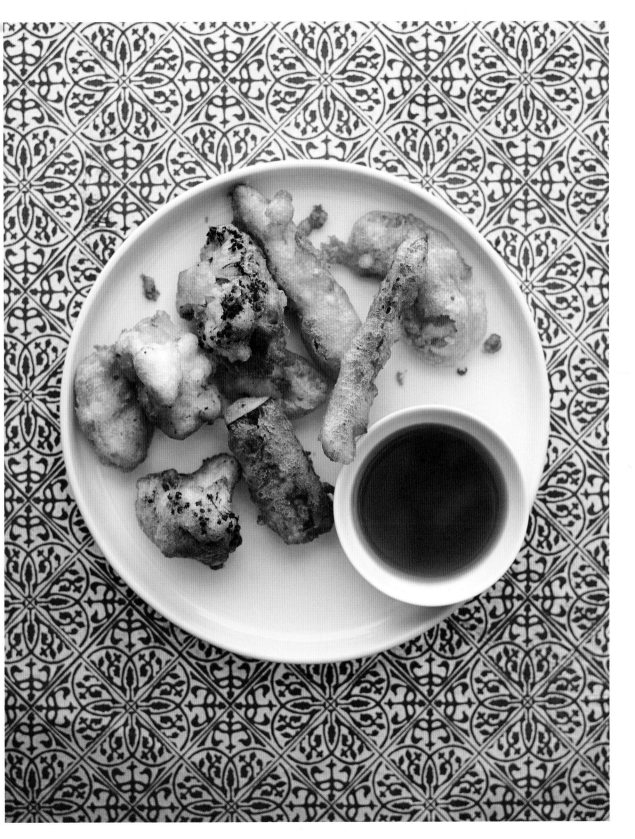

SPICED INVOLTINI PRIMAVERA | *serves 2 (makes 4)*

We have given these Italian rolls an Indian makeover with the addition of curry spices and paneer cheese. Perfect for a light lunch, or as a snack.

1 tbsp sunflower oil
½ tsp medium-hot curry powder
¼ tsp ground cumin
pinch of chilli powder
1 garlic clove, crushed
4 fine asparagus spears, cut in 6cm lengths
50g paneer cheese, cut into 4 strips
1 small aubergine, sliced lengthways in 5mm strips (you'll need 4 strips)
1 courgette, sliced lengthways in 5mm strips (again, you'll need 4 strips)
4 spring onions, green parts only, cut into long thin strips (optional)

2 OF YOUR 5-A-DAY

Preheat the grill to a medium setting.

Prepare the marinade by mixing the oil, curry powder, cumin, chilli powder and garlic. Brush the asparagus, paneer and both sides of the aubergine and courgette slices with the marinade. Place the aubergine and courgette slices under the grill for 10 minutes, being careful not to let them burn. Turn over the strips, add the asparagus and paneer and grill for a further 10 minutes until everything has softened, but the aubergine and courgette still retain their structure.

Leave to cool for 10 minutes. Make four individual rolls by placing each courgette slice on top of an aubergine slice, then place one-quarter of the asparagus and paneer at one end and roll up. Finally, tie with the spring onion, if using. Repeat to make four rolls.

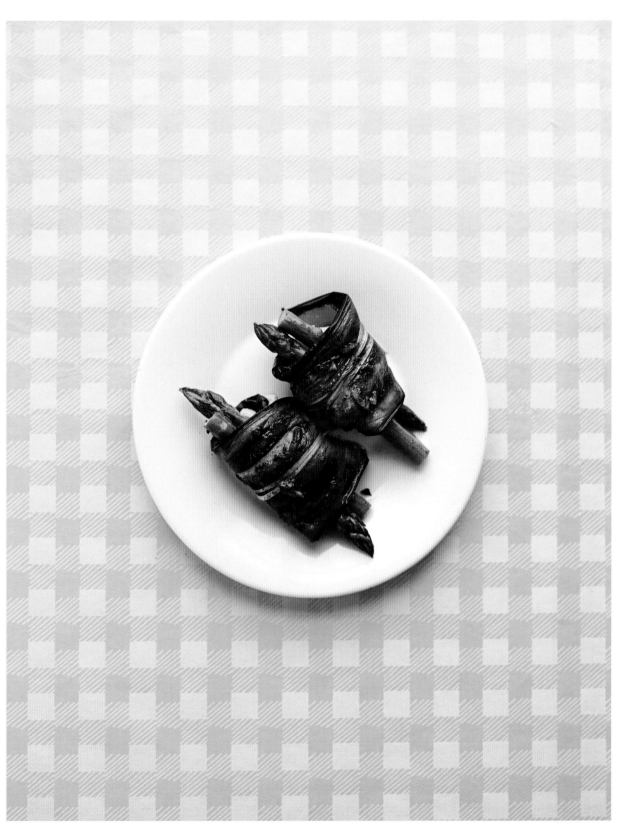

CUCUMBER AND HOUMOUS MAKI | *serves 4 (makes 20 pieces)*

A very simple but healthy snack, these cucumber bites can be filled with many of our dips (see pages 164–181) to make a colourful plate of refreshing nibbles. Our North African-spiced houmous with roasted red pepper adds a portion of vegetables to the traditional recipe, as well as being lighter and more colourful.

1 large cucumber (320g)

For the red pepper houmous
1 red pepper (160g)
400g can of chickpeas, drained, but reserve the liquid from the can
1 large garlic clove, crushed
1 tbsp tahini
1 tbsp extra virgin olive oil
juice of ½ lemon
1 heaped tsp ras-el-hanout
sea salt and freshly ground black pepper

2 OF YOUR 5-A-DAY

To make the houmous, put the red pepper under a hot grill, turning as the skin blackens and blisters. Once the skin has been charred all over, put the pepper in a bowl and cover with cling film. When cool, remove the skin and deseed.

Put the flesh of the red pepper and the drained chickpeas in a food processor with the crushed garlic. Add 1 tbsp of the chickpea liquid, the tahini, olive oil, lemon juice and ras-el-hanout. Process until smooth. Season with salt and pepper.

Top and tail the cucumber. Cut into four equal pieces, then cut each piece into five rounds. Scoop out a few of the seeds from each round to make room for the filling, but be careful not to make a hole through to the bottom. Add 1 heaped tsp of houmous to each slice of cucumber. There will be some left over, but pop it in an airtight container in the fridge and use another time (it will keep for three days and you will have used it all up as a dip well before then).

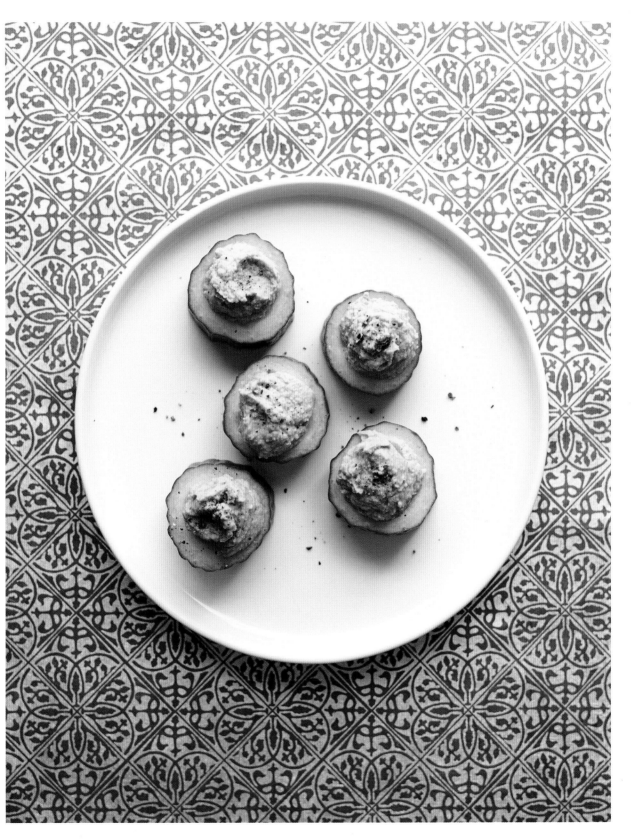

MINTED PEA AND PEPPER NORI | *serves 2 (makes 12 pieces)*

Our version of this healthy Japanese snack omits rice but uses nori sheets with dips and raw vegetables instead. This recipe uses a minted pea filling with red pepper, but experiment with your own creative and colourful combinations. Gorgeous guacamole (see page 174) with carrot is another favourite.

For the minted pea filling
1 tbsp vegetable oil
2 banana shallots, finely chopped (80g)
sea salt and freshly ground black pepper
160g frozen petit pois
small handful of mint leaves

For the rest
2 nori sheets
½ red pepper, cut into thin 10cm-long batons (80g)

2 OF YOUR 5-A-DAY

Heat the oil in a heavy-based saucepan. Fry the shallots over a medium heat for about five minutes until translucent. Season lightly with salt and pepper.

Add the peas and 2 tbsp of water, followed by the mint. Cook for one or two minutes before placing in a blender. Blend to a coarse-textured purée.

Cut each nori sheet in half to create four rectangular shapes each about 20 x 10cm. Make sure your hands are very dry, as the sheets easily soften. With the shiny side facing down, position one of the rectangles with the short side in front of you. From the bottom of the rectangle, spread one-quarter of the filling three-quarters of the way up the sheet, leaving a 3cm gap at the top edge (this stops the filling squeezing out when you go to bite it).

Place one-quarter of the red pepper batons at the bottom of the rectangle and roll up. Wet the gap with your finger to ensure the nori sticks. Repeat with the other sheets and filling.

With a sharp knife, cut each roll into three. Serve.

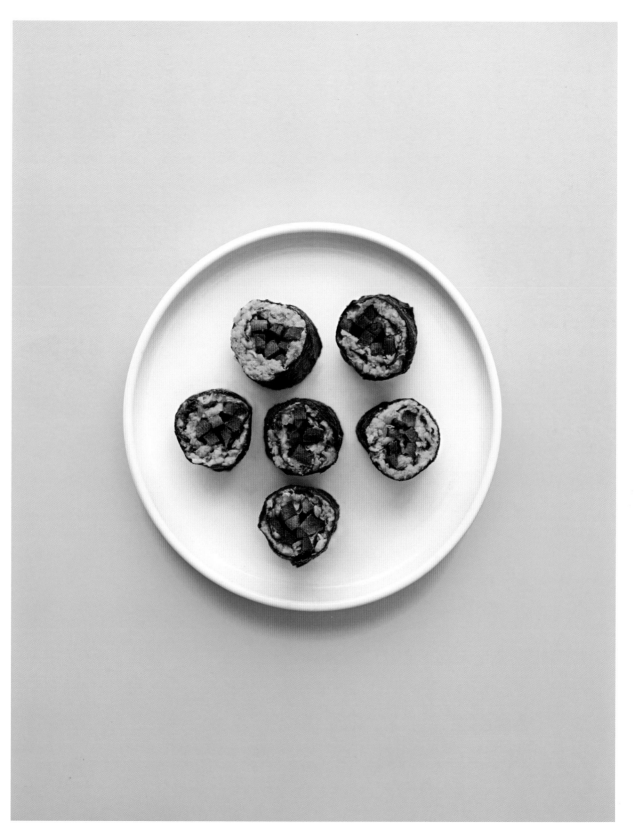

CARROT TZATZIKI | *serves 2*

A really light, refreshing dip and extremely easy to make. Our tzatziki recipe uses carrot and cumin as well as cucumber to make an unusual but really colourful and tasty dip.

300g Greek yogurt
1 medium carrot, coarsely grated (80g)
¼ cucumber, deseeded and
grated (80g)
2 garlic cloves, crushed
large handful of mint leaves,
finely chopped
finely grated zest and juice of
1 unwaxed lemon
½ tsp ground cumin
1 tbsp olive oil
sea salt and freshly
ground black pepper
crudités or warm pitta breads,
to serve

1 OF YOUR 5-A-DAY

Place the yogurt, carrot, cucumber, garlic and mint into a bowl. Add the lemon zest and sprinkle over the cumin. Mix well and finish with some lemon juice, olive oil, salt and pepper to taste.

Serve with crudités or warm pitta.

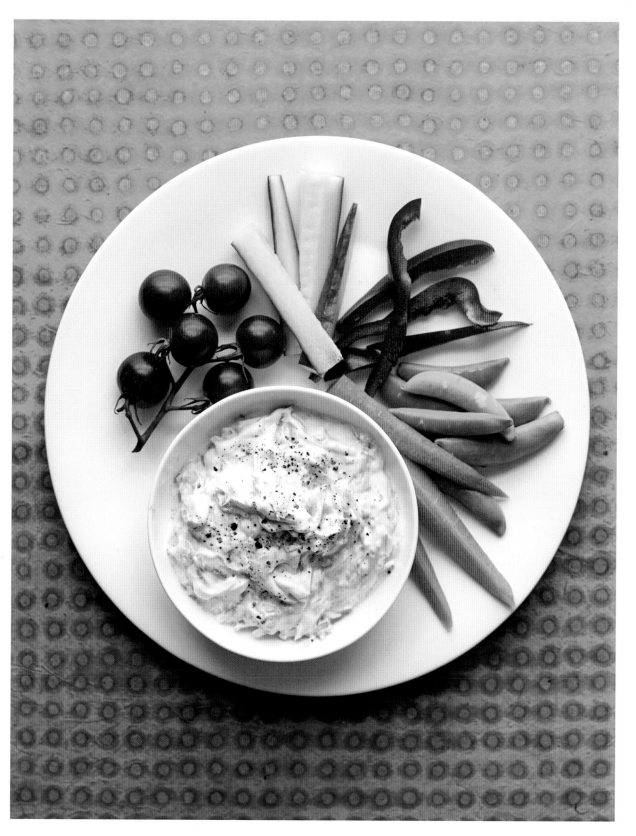

TOMATO, AVOCADO AND MANGO SALSA | *serves 4*

Great as a dip, or – chopped more coarsely – a really vibrant and chunky salad to accompany fish or meat. If you like a hotter salsa, substitute jalapeño peppers for the green pepper.

1 small ripe mango (160g)
2 large tomatoes (160g)
1 avocado (160g)
½ green pepper (80g), or 2–3 jalapeños
   if you like it hot
1 small red onion (80g)
1 red chilli, deseeded
1 tbsp finely chopped mint leaves
2 tbsp finely chopped coriander
sea salt and freshly ground black pepper
juice of 1 lime
1 tbsp extra virgin olive oil (optional)
a few basil leaves, torn,
   to serve

2 OF YOUR 5-A-DAY

Cut off the mango 'cheeks' on either side of the large seed and cut a criss-cross pattern in each. Turn each half inside out, then cut off the cubes of flesh.

Chop the mango, tomatoes, avocado and green pepper finely if you want a salsa, or more coarsely if you want a salad.

Finely chop the onion and chilli.

Mix everything together with the mint and coriander and season with salt, pepper, lime juice and oil (if using).

Finish with the torn basil leaves.

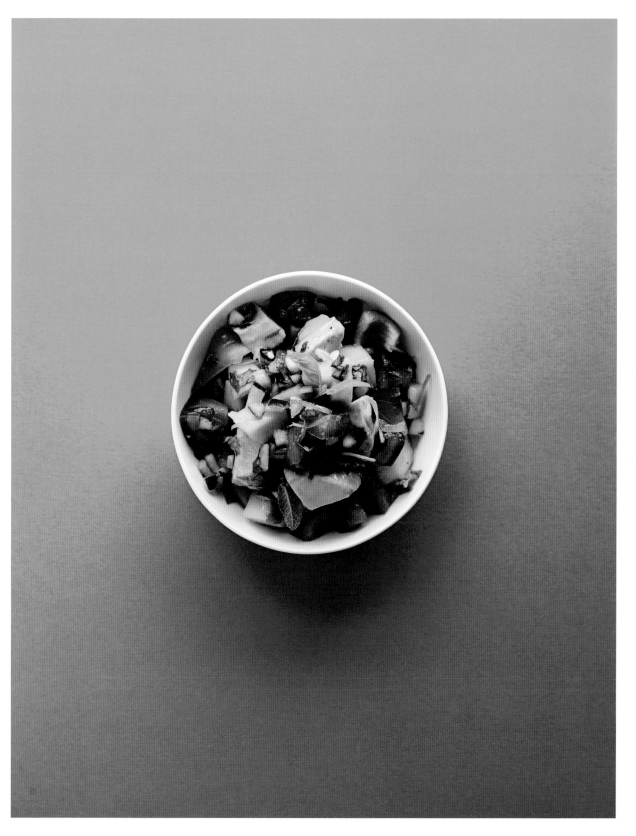

BABA GHANOUSH | *serves 4*

This Middle Eastern aubergine dip is enhanced with sumac and red onion, giving an extra twist. Lovely with warm pitta bread as a starter or snack.

2 large red onions, quartered (320g)
1 garlic clove, skin on
1 tbsp sunflower oil
1 large aubergine (400g)
2 tbsp extra virgin olive oil, plus more to serve (optional)
1 heaped tsp tahini
good squeeze of lemon juice
1 tsp sumac
handful of chopped parsley leaves
sea salt and freshly ground black pepper

2 OF YOUR 5-A-DAY

Preheat the oven to 200°C/fan 180°C/400°F/gas mark 6.

Toss the onions and unpeeled garlic clove on a baking tray with the sunflower oil. Place the whole aubergine on the same tray and roast for about 45 minutes to one hour.

Once the aubergine has cooked and collapsed, scoop out the soft flesh (discarding the skin) and place in a food processor. Remove the outer skin from the roasted garlic and add to the aubergine, together with the roasted onions. Add the extra virgin olive oil, tahini, lemon juice, sumac, parsley and salt and pepper. Blend until everything is smooth.

Place in a bowl and drizzle a little more extra virgin olive oil over the top (if required) before serving.

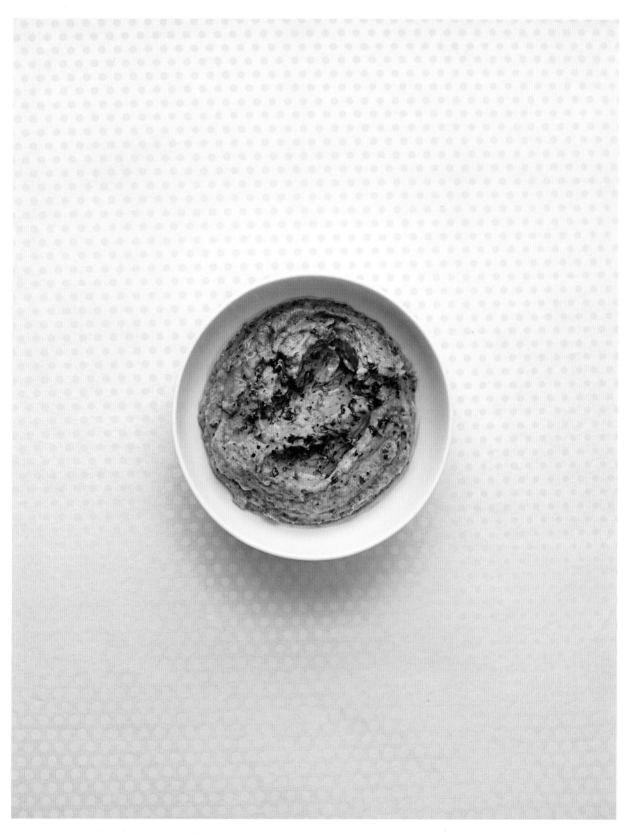

CUCUMBER AND BANANA RAITA | *serves 4*

This may sound like an odd combination and we were certainly all sceptical when our head chef, Neel, recommended it. But it's a fantastic mixture, plus it ups your five-a-day in a really easy way.

1 small cucumber (240g)
1 small banana (80g)
2 tbsp finely chopped coriander
2 tbsp finely chopped mint leaves
300g natural yogurt
juice of ½ lemon
pinch of chilli powder
sea salt

1 OF YOUR 5-A-DAY

Deseed the cucumber and chop it very finely (leaving the skin on).

Peel the banana and mash with a fork.

Mix the cucumber, banana and herbs into the yogurt and season with the lemon juice, chilli powder and salt to taste.

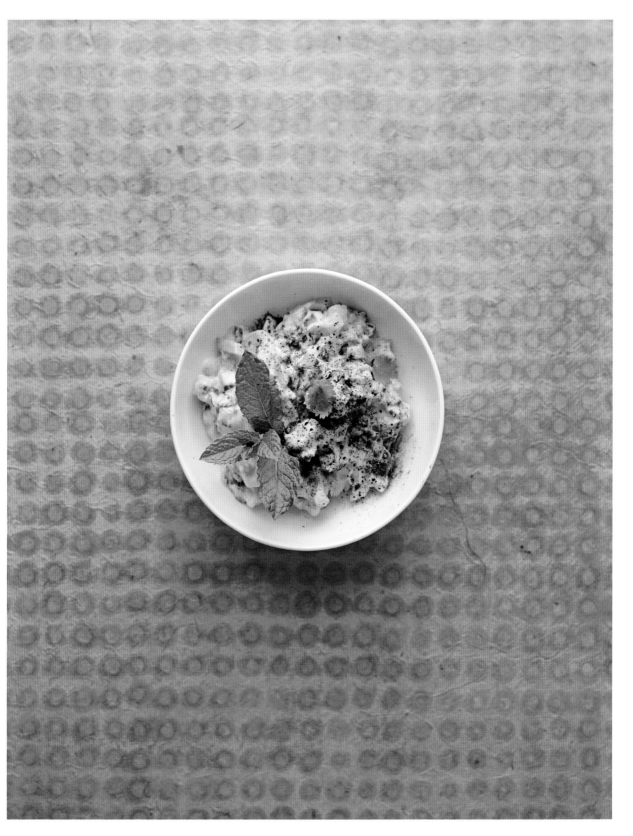

CHUNKY COURGETTE, PEPPER AND CHILLI SALSA | *serves 2*

A really fresh, spicy vegetable salsa with so much more flavour than most shop-bought varieties. Made with a combination of green and red chillies and peppers, this salsa is very colourful and is great to eat with corn chips, or crudités if you are feeling more virtuous.

4–5 large tomatoes, peeled or not as
   you prefer, chopped (320g)
½ green pepper, chopped (80g)
½ red pepper, chopped (80g)
½ courgette, finely chopped (80g)
½ medium onion, chopped (80g)
1 green jalapeño chilli pepper, deseeded
   and finely chopped (leave the seeds in
   if you like it hot)
1 red chilli pepper, deseeded and finely
   chopped (again, leave the seeds in if
   you like it hot)
4 tbsp white wine vinegar
1 tsp caster sugar
1 garlic clove, finely chopped
½ tsp ground cumin
½ tsp sea salt
¼ tsp dried oregano
¼ tsp Tabasco sauce (optional)
handful of chopped coriander
corn chips or crudités, to serve

**3 OF YOUR
5-A-DAY**

Combine all the ingredients in a medium-sized saucepan and bring to the boil.

Reduce the heat and simmer, uncovered, stirring frequently, for about 40 minutes, until slightly thickened.

With a hand-held blender, give the mixture a few quick blends, but ensure you keep the chunkiness of the salsa.

Let the salsa cool, then put it into a jar and refrigerate (this will keep for up to three days in the fridge).

Serve with corn chips or crudités.

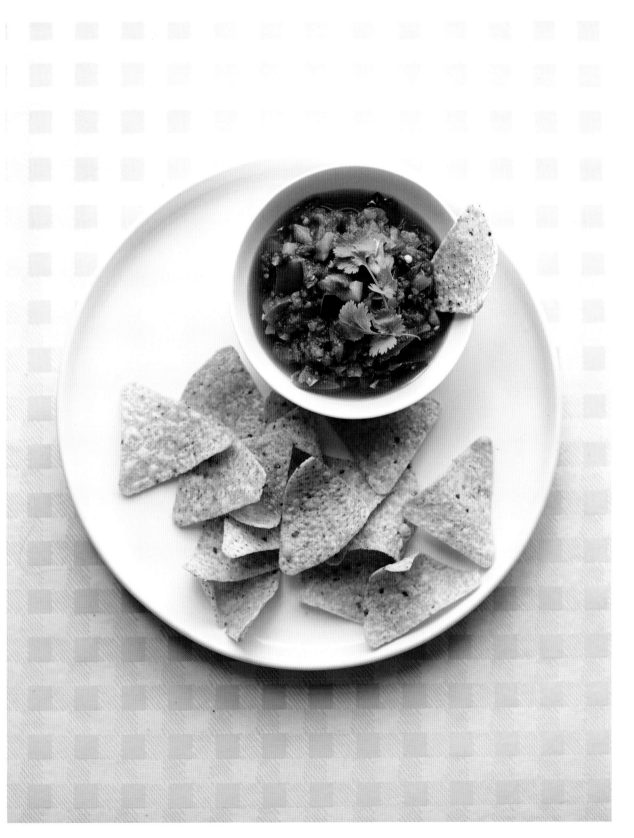

GORGEOUS GUACAMOLE *serves 2*

The subtle flavours of this luxurious and creamy dip have been given a kick in our version with the addition of chilli and lime. The red onion and tomato give it more substance, a little crunch and a great colour.

1 large ripe avocado (160g)
1 large tomato, deseeded and finely chopped (80g)
1 small red onion, finely chopped (80g)
1 red or green chilli, finely chopped (optional)
1 tbsp chopped coriander
1 tsp finely chopped parsley leaves (optional)
1 tbsp extra virgin olive oil
sea salt and freshly ground black pepper
juice of 1 lime, or to taste

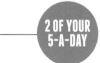

2 OF YOUR 5-A-DAY

Mash the avocado with a fork and mix in the tomato, red onion and chilli, if using.

Mix in the coriander and parsley (if using) and season with extra virgin olive oil, salt, pepper and plenty of lime juice.

Top Tip: This makes a great filler for pitta pockets, wraps or our Nori rolls (see page 162). Alternatively, place a flour tortilla in a dry frying pan, spread over the guacamole with a sprinkling of grated cheese and fold over to form a semi-circle. Fry on both sides for a couple of minutes until golden brown and the cheese has melted.

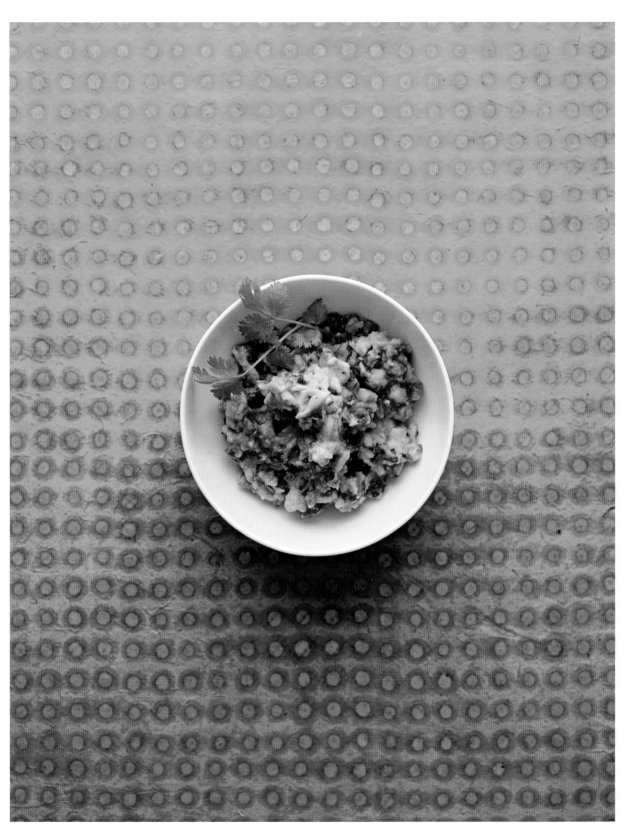

CHILLI SAMBAL | *serves 2*

This hot and spicy all-purpose accompaniment originates from Indonesia. It can be added to any kind of dish to provide an extra kick: soups, stews, rice or noodles. It is traditionally made in a mortar and pestle, giving a wonderful aroma as you grind the ingredients, but a blender works perfectly well if you are pushed for time.

6 long hot red chillies, cayenne
   are ideal
5 garlic cloves
1 tsp finely chopped root ginger
2 banana shallots, finely chopped (80g)
6 kaffir lime leaves, stems removed,
   leaves shredded
1 lemon grass stalk, tough outer leaves
   removed, finely chopped
2 tbsp flavourless vegetable oil
1 tbsp palm sugar
1 tsp salt
2 tbsp lime juice

**1 OF YOUR
5-A-DAY**

Put the chillies, garlic, ginger, shallots, lime leaves and lemon grass into a blender and blend to form a paste, adding a little water to help it along, if necessary.

Heat the oil in a heavy-based saucepan and sauté the chilli paste over a medium heat, being careful not to burn it. Reduce the heat and simmer for five minutes before adding the sugar and salt. Continue stirring until the mixture becomes darker.

Remove from the heat and leave to cool. Stir in the lime juice to brighten the flavours, then serve.

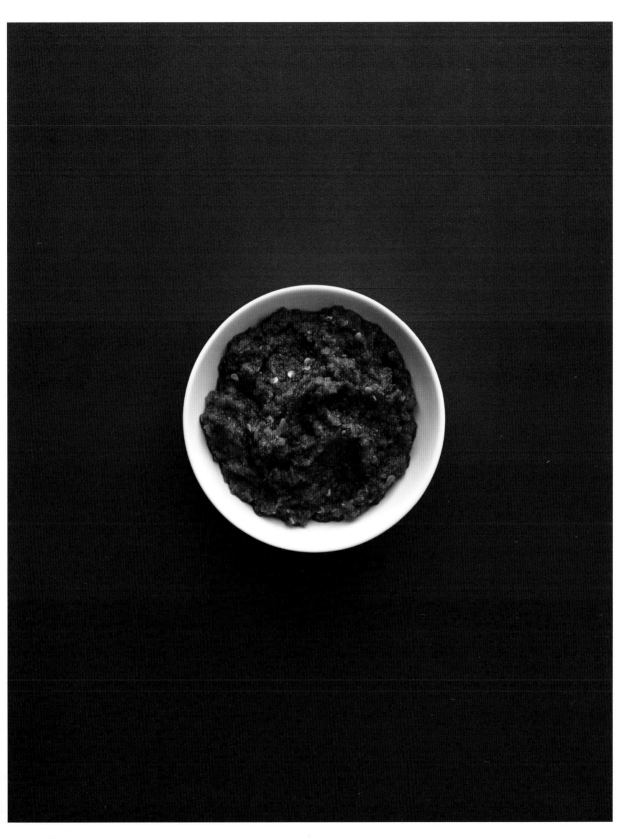

PINEAPPLE CHUTNEY | *serves 2*

Surprise your guests with this tangy, chunky condiment. The smell of spices will fill your home as you reduce this exotic mix to a sticky, spicy chutney. Delicious as an alternative to mango chutney to serve with poppadums or spicy curries.

1 tbsp sunflower oil
1 cinnamon stick
1 tsp cumin seeds
1 tsp mustard seeds
sprig of curry leaves (leave out if you
   can't find fresh leaves)
1 small onion, finely chopped (80g)
1 heaped tsp grated root ginger
1 red chilli, finely chopped
1 tsp ground turmeric
2 tbsp cider vinegar
1 tbsp caster sugar
230g can of pineapple pieces in
   fruit juice, drained (or the
   equivalent weight of fresh
   pineapple, chopped)

1 OF YOUR 5-A-DAY

Heat the oil in a heavy-based saucepan and add the cinnamon stick followed by the cumin seeds, mustard seeds and curry leaves. Fry for about 30 seconds, or until the seeds start to change colour and pop.

Add the onion and cook for two minutes before adding the ginger and chilli. Cook for a further two minutes before adding the turmeric.

Add the vinegar, sugar, pineapple and 175ml of water and simmer for just over one hour, stirring from time to time.

The chutney will keep in the fridge, in an airtight container, for up to one week.

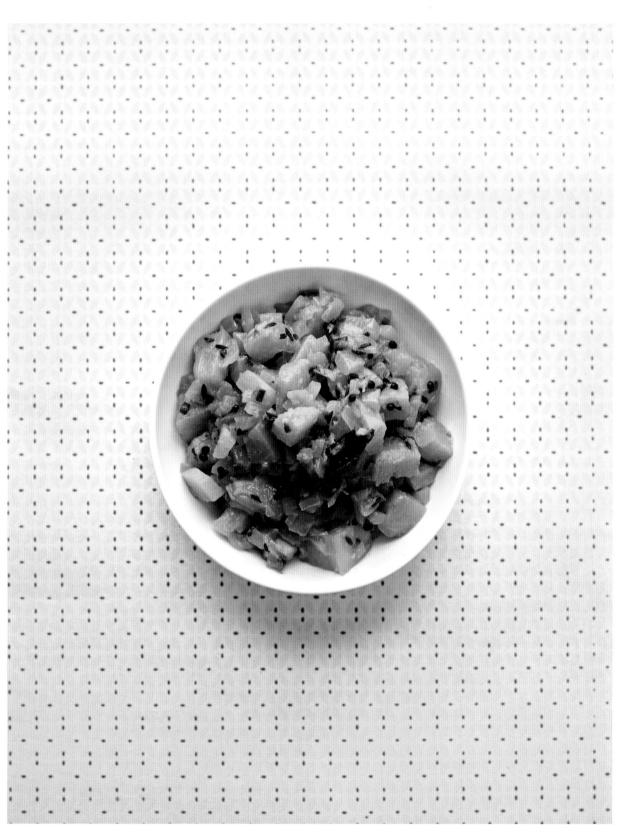

SIMPLE CHILLI SAUCE | *serves 4*

A very versatile chilli dip which gives you another portion of your five-a-day while spicing up any kind of snack. Alternatively add a tablespoon or two to any dish to give it an extra kick.

4 large tomatoes
2 tsp tomato purée
1 tbsp tomato ketchup
1 green chilli, finely chopped
½ small onion, finely chopped
2 tbsp finely chopped coriander
½ tsp cumin seeds
½ tsp ground cumin
good squeeze of lemon juice
sea salt

1 OF YOUR 5-A-DAY

Score a cross in the base of each tomato, then place in a bowl and cover with some boiling water. Leave for two minutes before draining and slipping off the skins. Remove the seeds from the tomatoes and blitz with the purée and ketchup in a small food processor.

Stir the chilli, onion and coriander into the tomato mixture with the cumin seeds, ground cumin, lemon juice and salt.

This keeps in the fridge for three days in an airtight container.

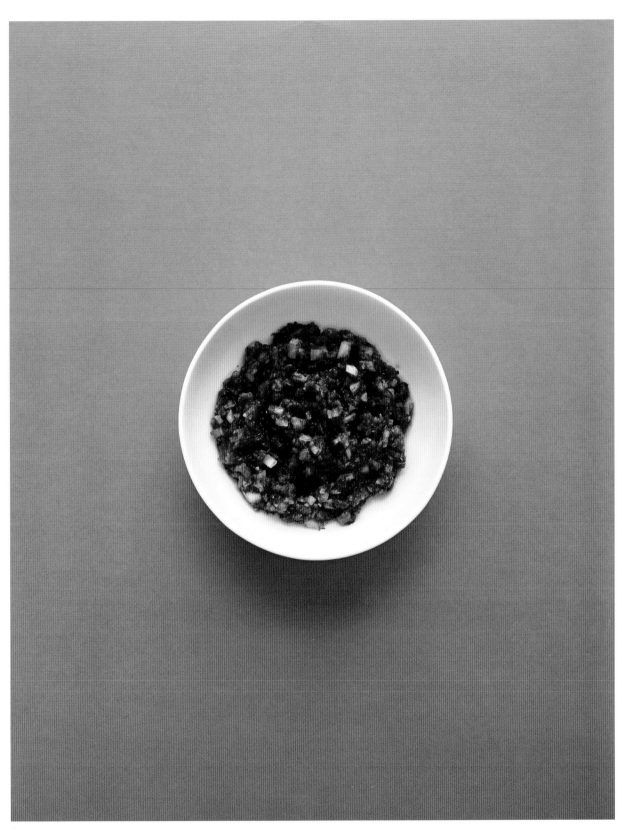

TOP UP YOUR 5: DESSERTS

Fruit is sweet, refreshing and easy to eat and should be included in a balanced diet. While fresh fruit on its own often makes a perfect dessert, sometimes something slightly 'naughtier' is called for. The tempting and delicious desserts in this chapter will be hard to resist, and will give you up to two portions of your five-a-day. Needless to say, they are recommended as occasional treats only!

STRAWBERRY, ELDERFLOWER AND APPLE JELLIES | *serves 2*

Taking inspiration from the English summer garden, this dessert is really light and refreshing. Sensual flavours hide its simplicity, as it uses only a few fresh ingredients. To add an exotic crunch we use pistachio nuts, but it works equally well with a light sprinkling of finely chopped mint leaves.

1 large dessert apple (such as Gala),
   peeled, cored and cubed
3 tbsp elderflower cordial
175ml apple and elderflower juice
10 large or 14 medium
   strawberries (160g)
½ sachet (6g) powdered gelatine
chopped pistachios, to serve

2 OF YOUR 5-A-DAY

Place the apple in a small pan with the elderflower cordial and the apple and elderflower juice. Bring to the boil and simmer for five minutes.

Retain your two prettiest strawberries for decoration and quarter the rest. Add the chopped strawberries to the apple mix and continue to cook for one minute. This will give your liquid a lovely pink colour. Strain out the fruit and set aside, then return the juices to the pan.

Heat the liquid gently, sprinkle on the gelatine and whisk vigorously until fully dissolved.

Divide the apple and strawberries between two serving dishes and pour the jelly evenly over the fruit.

Put in the fridge for about 45 minutes to set. Serve with the reserved strawberries on top and sprinkled with pistachios.

Top Tip: Try this with elderflower liqueur instead of cordial

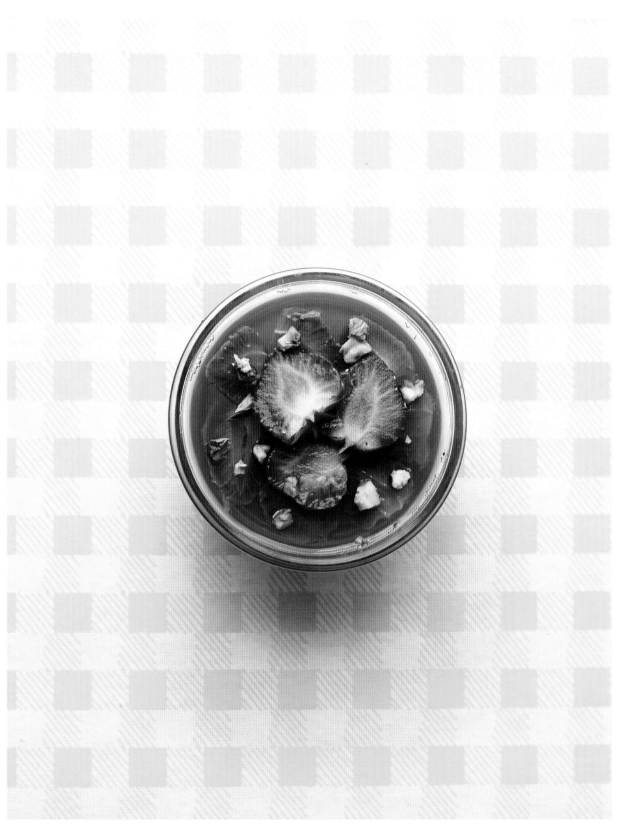

SPICED PEARS AND PLUMS
IN RED WINE SYRUP | *serves 4*

The scent of star anise and cardamom will fill your home as you prepare this delicious dish. Although reminiscent of dark winter nights, this sweet and tangy combination is the perfect way to end a meal on a summer's evening. It's also an easy recipe to prepare in advance.

4 Conference pears
6 plums
1 vanilla pod
1 bottle of red wine
100g soft brown sugar
1 cinnamon stick
1 star anise
2 tsp ground cardamom
200g fromage frais

**2 OF YOUR
5-A-DAY**

Peel the pears but keep them whole with the stalks intact. Quarter the plums and remove the stones.

Halve the vanilla pod lengthways and scrape out the black seeds. Cut each piece of pod into three long thin strips and add to a saucepan with the seeds, the wine, sugar, cinnamon stick, star anise and cardamom. Use a slotted spoon to lower in the pears.

Poach over a gentle heat for 30–40 minutes, making sure the pears are covered with the wine. The cooking time will depend on the ripeness of your pears; they should be tender all the way through when pierced with a cocktail stick. You can make these up to two days ahead and chill.

Remove the pears from the pan, add the quartered plums to the liquid and bring to the boil. After two to three minutes, remove the plums and continue to reduce the liquid by half so that it becomes syrupy (about 20–30 minutes). Strain the syrup, but retain the vanilla and cinnamon.

Serve each pear surrounded by roughly 6 pieces of plum with the cooled syrup, a strip of vanilla, a piece of cinnamon and dollop of fromage frais.

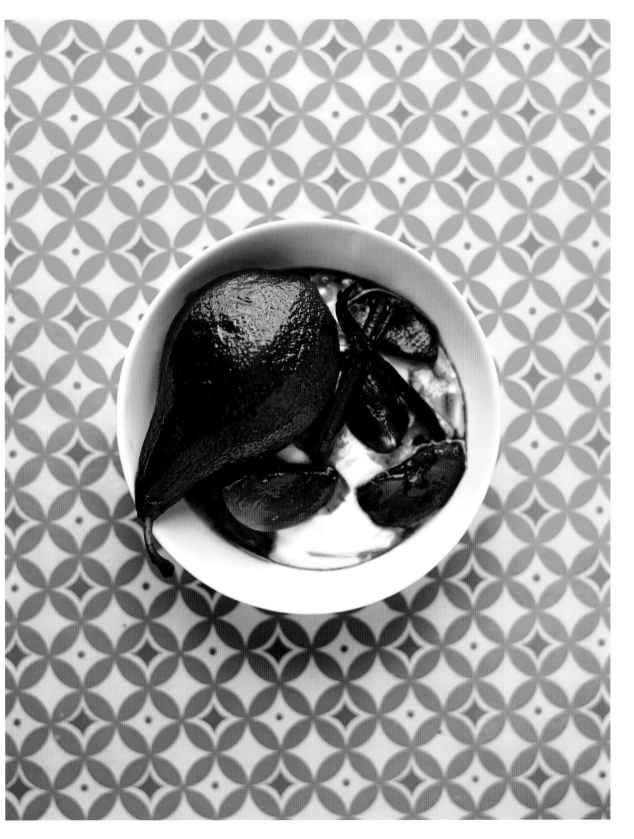

EXOTIC ETON MESS | *serves 2*

Our Eton Mess recipe is inspired by Eastern cuisine, combining sweet mango and blueberries with a pomegranate jus and a passion fruit cream. This dessert is as gorgeous to look at as it is to eat, and topping the Mess with pomegranate and passion fruit seeds provides freshness and crunch.

1 pomegranate
1 tbsp caster sugar
1 small ripe mango (160g)
1 large passion fruit
100ml whipping cream
1 punnet of blueberries (160g)
1 regular-sized meringue

2 OF YOUR 5-A-DAY

Deseed the pomegranate by placing it curved side up over a bowl and bashing the skin of the halved fruit with a large spoon. Retain a small handful of seeds and place the rest in a pan with the sugar. Heat until you can extract all the juice by mashing with a potato masher, then strain and set aside.

Cut off the mango 'cheeks' on either side of the large seed and cut a criss-cross pattern in each. Turn each half inside out, then cut off the cubes of flesh.

Halve the passion fruit and scoop the seeds into a bowl.

Whisk the cream until stiff. Add the juice from the passion fruit and half the passion fruit seeds to the cream and mix fully. Stir in half the mango and half the blueberries.

Assemble the dessert by dividing the remaining mango and blueberries between two serving dishes. Crumble half the meringue over the fruit and pour the pomegranate juice over.

Scoop the fruity cream mix on top. Crumble over the remaining meringue and sprinkle with the remaining passion fruit and pomegranate seeds.

Serve immediately.

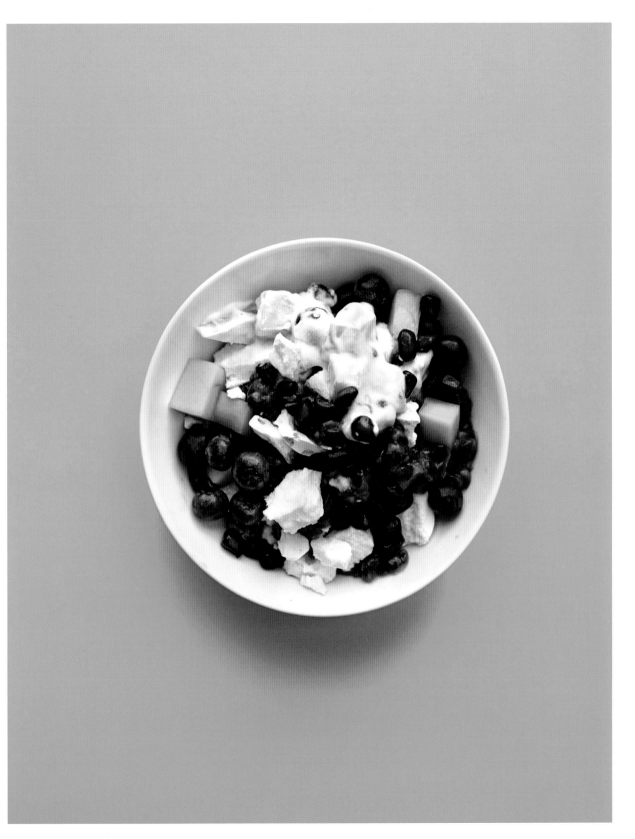

SUMMER PUDDING WITH LAVENDER CREAM | *serves 4*

There is something wonderful about this quintessentially British dessert. Enclosing a medley of seasonal fruit, the bread dome is sealed with a jam lining, creating a beautifully marbled effect. This dish is ideally prepared the night before serving. For a lighter pudding with the same flavours, try our Summer berry compôte (see page 192).

*flavourless vegetable oil or unsalted
   butter, for the basin*
*640g mixed summer berries
   (raspberries, redcurrants, strawberries,
   blackcurrants, blackberries), stalks
   removed, strawberries hulled
   and quartered*
100g caster sugar
1 tbsp rose water
juice of ½ orange
½ tsp vanilla bean paste (optional)
*3 tsp low-sugar blackcurrant
   jam (optional)*
*6 thin slices from a large white loaf,
   crusts removed*
110ml whipping cream
4–5 lavender flower heads

**2 OF YOUR
5-A-DAY**

Oil or butter a 850ml pudding basin, then line with two sheets of cling film, leaving a 3–4cm overhang.

Place all the berries in a large, heavy-based saucepan with the sugar, rose water, orange juice and vanilla bean paste (if using). Cook over a low heat for three to five minutes, until the sugar dissolves and juices start bleeding from the fruit. Turn off the heat and leave in the pan.

Spread the jam over the bread; it will block the seepage of the juices and add to the final marbled effect, so leave it out if you would prefer a more homogenous appearance. Line the basin with five of the slices, jam facing inside, overlapping slightly to ensure no gaps and pressing the bread against the sides.

Spoon the fruit and half its juice into the basin. Cover the pudding with the last slice of bread, then pull over the overhanging cling film. Place a saucer that fits inside the basin on top, then place a weight, about 2kg, on top of that. Refrigerate overnight to soak up the juices.

Strain the leftover juice through a fine sieve into a small pan. Bring to the boil, then simmer for five to 10 minutes, until reduced to a light syrup. Pour into a jug, cover and chill.

Heat the cream gently but do not bring to the boil. Add the lavender heads. Cover and chill overnight to infuse. Next day, remove the lavender and whip the cream to stiff peaks.

To serve, unwrap the cling film and carefully invert the pudding on to a plate. Now you must take a view: you can use the berry juices to 'paint' any white area, or leave the pudding marbled and drizzle the juice over the cream.

Either way, serve with a dollop of fragrant lavender cream.

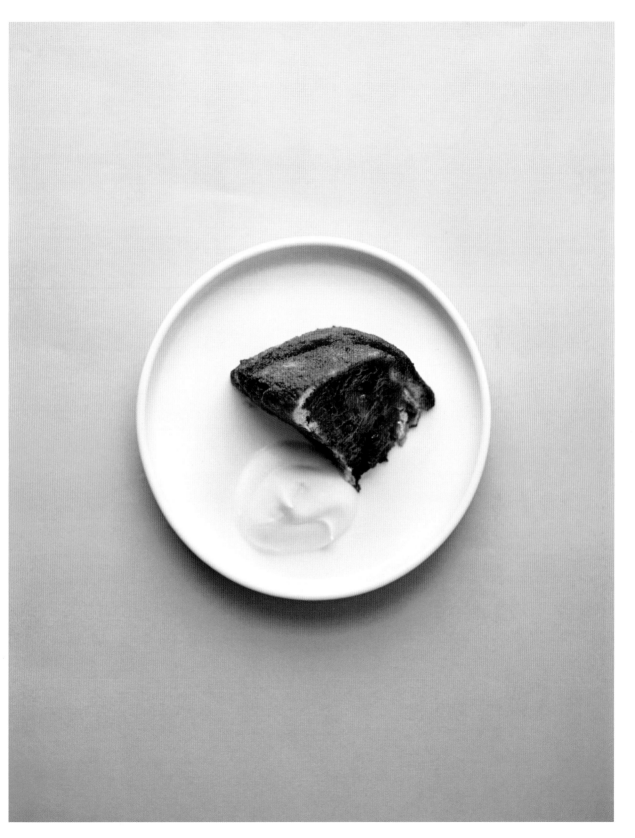

SUMMER BERRY COMPOTE WITH GREEK YOGURT | *serves 4*

This beautifully coloured dessert combines a medley of lightly cooked seasonal fruit with creamy Greek yogurt. This dish is ideally prepared the night before to allow the compôte to get really cold. It's also great for breakfast. To make a more composed dish with the same basic flavours, try the Summer pudding with lavender cream (see page 190).

640g mixed summer berries (raspberries, redcurrants, strawberries, blackcurrants, blackberries), stalks removed, strawberries hulled and quartered
50–80g soft brown sugar (depending on how sweet you like it)
1 tbsp rose water (optional)
juice of ½ orange
150ml Greek yogurt

2 OF YOUR 5-A-DAY

Place all the berries in a large, heavy-based saucepan with the sugar, rose water (if using) and orange juice. Cook over a low heat for five minutes, until the sugar dissolves and juices start bleeding from the fruit. Turn off the heat and leave in the pan to cool for 10 minutes.

Strain the berries through a fine sieve into a small pan. Set the berries aside. Bring the juice in the pan to the boil, then simmer for five to 10 minutes, until the juice has reduced to a light syrup. Pour into a jug, cover and keep in the fridge.

Serve the compôte with a dollop of creamy Greek yogurt and a drizzle of the syrup, which will have thickened overnight.

Top Tip: Any leftover juice makes a delicious summer fruit squash. Just add water in the ratio of 1:4 juice to water, and stir thoroughly to mix.

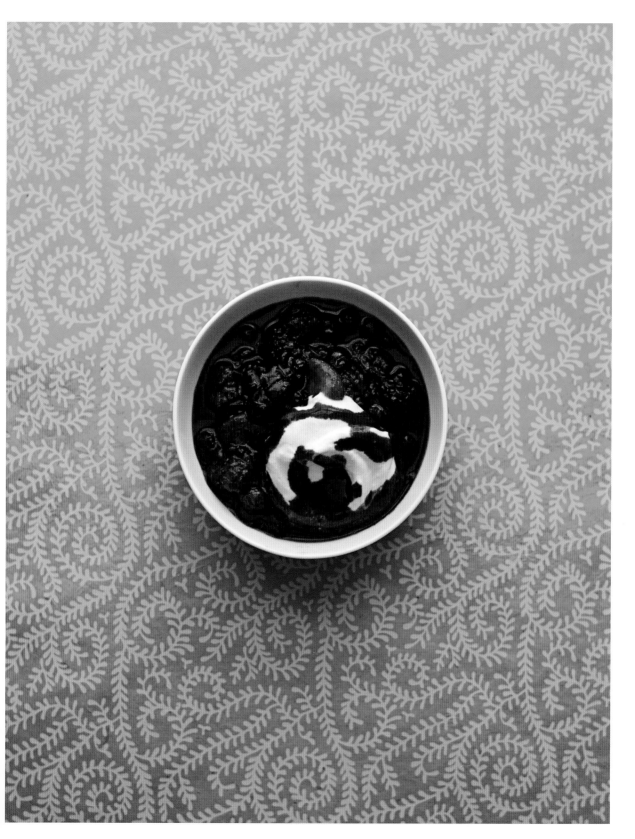

RHUBARB AND STRAWBERRY SORBET
WITH GINGER CREAM | *serves 4*

This dessert combines the refreshing zingy sweetness of rhubarb sorbet with a smooth, creamy, ginger-infused fromage frais. It is really quick to put together and can be made well in advance of serving.

320g rhubarb, chopped into small
    bite-sized pieces
320g strawberries, hulled and quartered
80g soft brown sugar
3 tbsp Chambord
2 tsp ginger jam
150g fromage frais

**2 OF YOUR
5-A-DAY**

Find a shallow metal freezerproof tray, about 20 x 10cm.

Place the rhubarb and strawberries in a heavy-based saucepan with the sugar and the liqueur. Heat over a medium-high heat for five minutes, then lower the heat and cook for a further 10 minutes to reduce the fruit mix.

Scoop it all into the shallow tray, leave to cool for 10 minutes, then place in the freezer for one or two hours. Scoop the frozen mixture into a bowl and beat it for two minutes to break the ice crystals and aerate the mixture.

At the same time, clean the metal tray and line it with cling film so that it overhangs by 3–5cm. Return the sorbet to the lined tray and re-freeze for one to two hours, or overnight.

Take the sorbet out of the freezer 20 minutes before serving. Now make the ginger cream by adding the ginger jam to the fromage frais and stirring thoroughly.

To serve, gently ease the sorbet out of the tin, place upside down on a clean chopping board and cut the sorbet into about 20 5 x 2cm strips, to mimic rhubarb sticks. Arrange the sorbet strips on a plate, add a dollop of ginger cream and serve immediately.

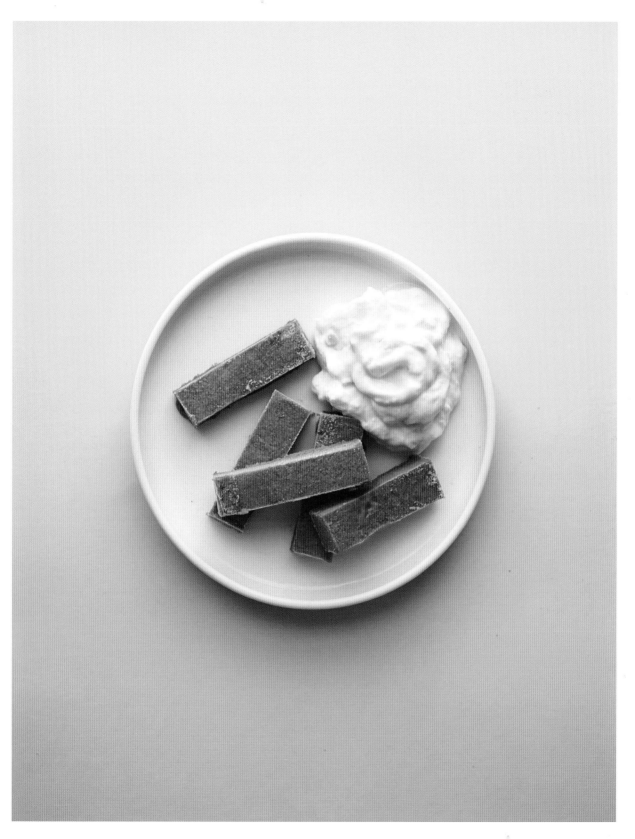

CHOCOLATE AND ORANGE CHICKPEA MOUSSE | *serves 4*

This mousse will surprise and delight you, so don't be put off by the inclusion of chickpeas! The dark chocolate and orange provide a rich flavour and texture.

400g can of chickpeas, drained and rinsed (net weight 240g)
150ml orange juice
150g dark chocolate
80g runny honey
2 tbsp Cointreau (optional)
3 small oranges (240g)
6g powdered gelatine
20 raspberries

2 OF YOUR 5-A-DAY

Place the chickpeas in a food processor and add the orange juice. Blend for three to four minutes until the mixture is as smooth as you can manage.

Melt the dark chocolate in a heatproof bowl over a pan of simmering water (the bowl must not touch the water). Pour the honey into the melting chocolate. Once fully melted, pour the chocolate mix into the food processor and add the Cointreau (if using). Blend for two minutes.

Remove the peel and pith from the oranges and slice them, taking care to remove any pips. Add to the food processor and blend again for a further two minutes.

Dissolve the gelatine in 50ml boiling water by whisking vigorously. Add to the food processor and blend for a final two minutes.

Divide the mixture between four 200ml ramekins and leave in the fridge for two or three hours to set.

Serve with five raspberries on each dish.

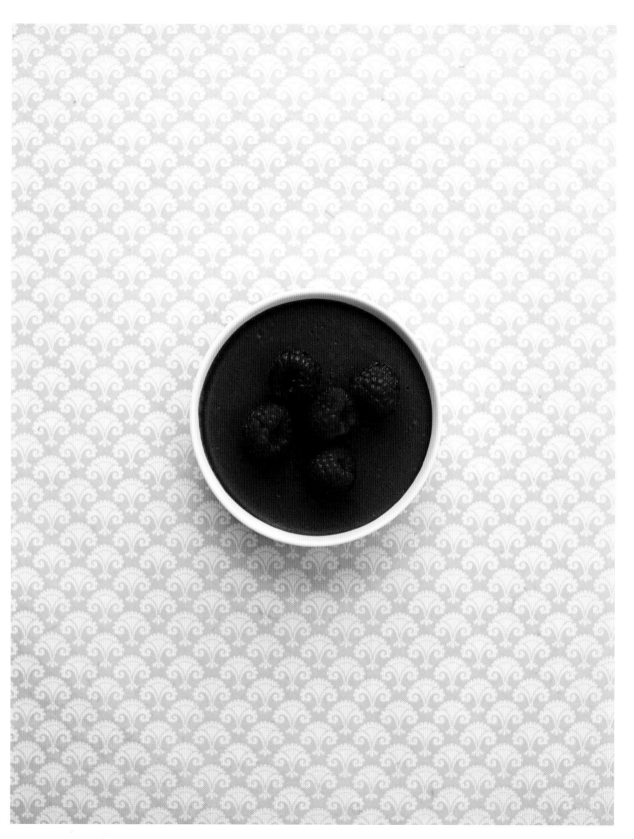

SPICED CARROT AND DATE MUFFINS | *makes 6*

These moist and delicately spiced muffins combine the sweetness of carrots, dates and sultanas with cinnamon and ginger spice. They are really easy to make and each muffin contains two portions of your five-a-day.

150g plain flour
pinch of salt
1 tsp baking powder
½ tsp bicarbonate of soda
60g soft brown sugar
1 tsp ground cinnamon
½ tsp ground ginger
360g carrots, coarsely grated
135g dates, finely chopped
90g sultanas
20g walnuts, finely chopped
1 egg, lightly beaten
90ml sunflower oil

2 OF YOUR 5-A-DAY

Preheat the oven to 200°C/fan 180°C/400°F/gas mark 6. Place six large muffin cases into a muffin tin.

Sift the flour, salt, baking powder and bicarbonate of soda into a mixing bowl. Stir in the sugar, cinnamon and ground ginger. Add the carrots, dates, sultanas and walnuts.

Add the egg to the mixture and pour in the oil. Mix quickly just until all the ingredients are combined. Divide evenly between the muffin cases until all the mixture is used and the cases are slightly over-filled. Push any exposed sultanas you can see down into the batter (they are more prone to burning).

Bake in the oven for 25–30 minutes or until well risen and golden brown. Ensure the muffins are cooked by testing with a skewer; it will come out clean when they are ready.

Lift out of the tin and leave to cool.

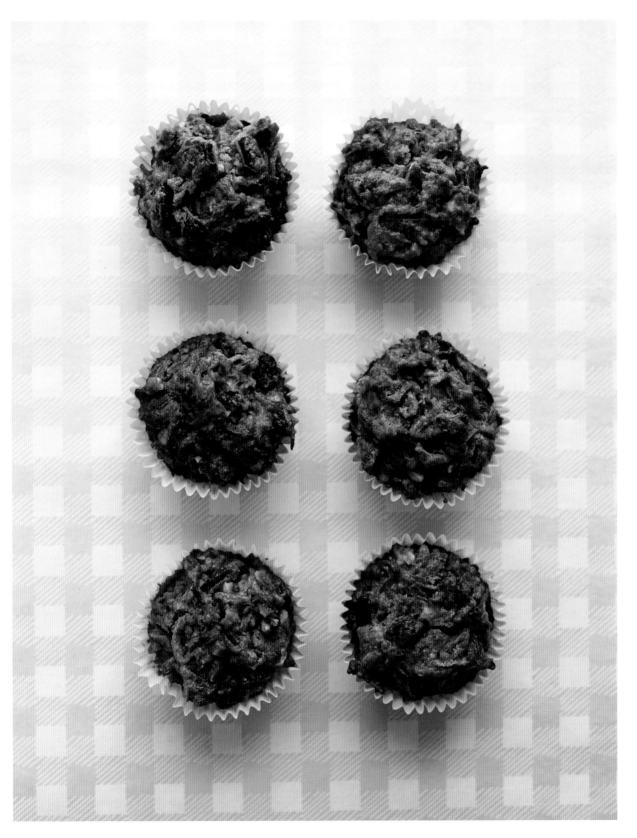

CARROT AND COURGETTE CAKE | *serves 8–10*

This moist and fruity celebration cake is a great alternative to a Christmas cake. With two portions of your five-a-day per slice, it combines a unique mix of courgette, carrot and banana, complemented by sweet raisins and apricots. No-one would ever guess how much goodness is in this cake!

150ml rapeseed oil, plus more for the tin
1 courgette (160g)
225g plain flour
2 tsp baking powder
1 tsp bicarbonate of soda
1 tsp sea salt
100g soft brown sugar
30g pine nuts, plus more for the top
120g raisins or sultanas
12 dried apricots, chopped
4 medium ripe bananas, mashed (320g)
3 eggs, lightly beaten
2 small carrots, grated (160g)

2 OF YOUR 5-A-DAY

Preheat the oven to 200°C/fan 180°C/400°F/gas mark 6. Oil a 23cm cake tin, preferably one with a springform base.

Grate the courgette. If it is very wet, let it drain for a short while in a colander or sieve, then press out excess moisture.

Sift the flour into a large bowl. Add the baking powder, bicarbonate of soda and salt. Mix in the sugar, pine nuts, raisins and apricots.

Add the bananas and eggs to the dry mix and stir, mixing in the grated carrots and courgette. Add the oil and beat thoroughly for one minute until you get a thick and slightly lumpy batter.

Spoon the batter into the prepared tin, sprinkle with a few more pine nuts and bake in the oven for 60 minutes, or until a skewer inserted into the centre comes out clean. Leave to stand for a few minutes before removing the cake from the tin. Make sure the cake is cold before slicing.

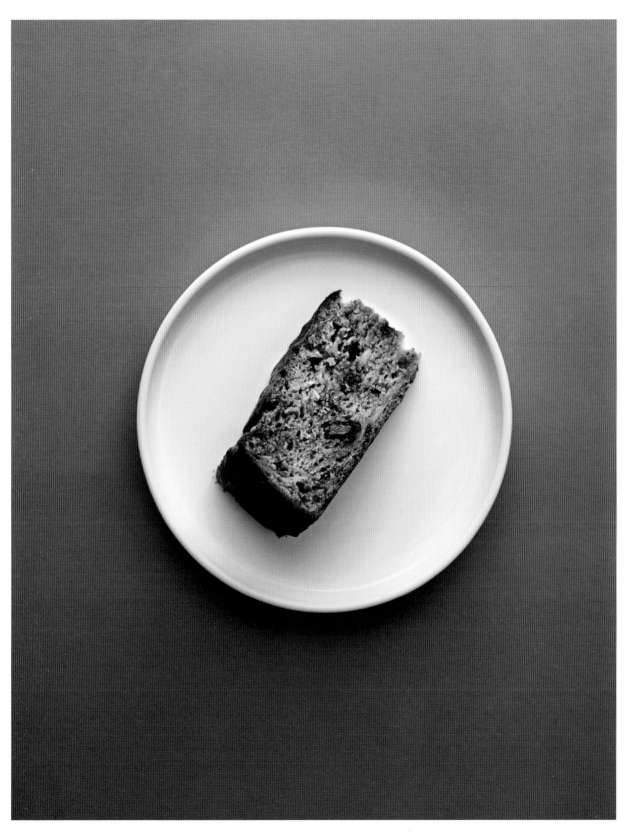

RAISIN AND APRICOT FLAPJACKS | *makes 8*

Classic flapjacks... but with a high fruit content. They look and smell delicious straight out of the oven, but resist the temptation to grab a slice until cool, as they need a little time to settle to keep their shape. The roasted pumpkin seeds add a delicious crunch. Apparently, they will store for up to four days in an airtight container... though in our house they have never made it beyond 24 hours.

20g pumpkin seeds
125g unsalted butter
50g soft brown sugar
2 tbsp set honey
175g oats
120g raisins
120g apricots, cut into
   raisin-sized pieces

1 OF YOUR 5-A-DAY

Preheat the oven to 200°C/fan 180°C/400°F/gas mark 6.

Dry-roast the pumpkin seeds in a pan for three to four minutes until they start to pop, then set aside.

Melt the butter, soft brown sugar and honey in a pan set over a low heat until the sugar is fully dissolved, about three minutes. Take care not to boil, and remove from the heat as soon as the sugar has fully dissolved. Add the oats, dried fruits and toasted pumpkin seeds and stir well.

Line a 15cm square cake tin with baking parchment and press the mixture into the tin, ensuring it fills the base completely and is level.

Score the cake into eight slices and bake for 25 minutes, or until golden brown.

Leave to cool in the tin for at least one hour. If any raisins have risen to the surface, press them back into the flapjack before leaving to cool. Once cooled, lift from the tin using the baking parchment to support the flapjack, then cut into bars, following the scored lines.

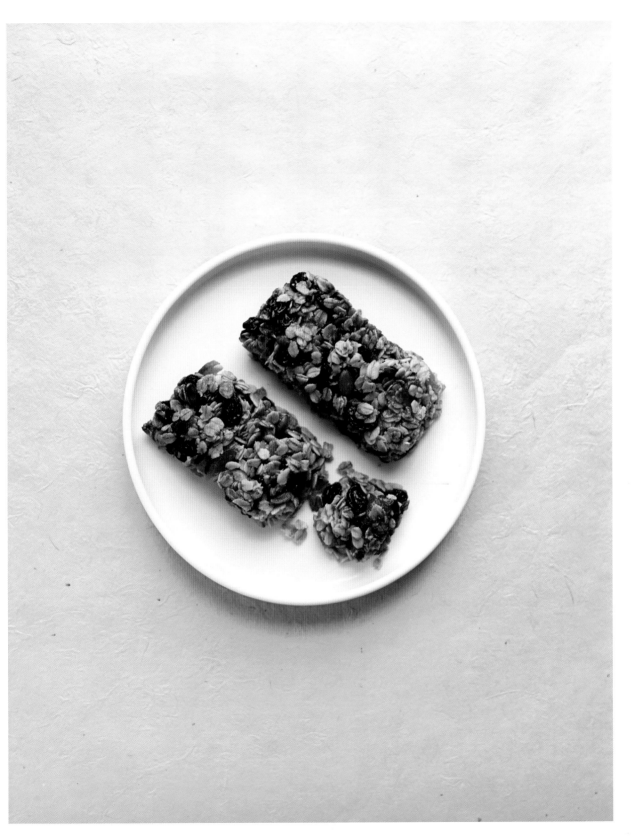

PINEAPPLE LOAF WITH FLAXSEED | *serves 10*

This is a really pretty cake that is excellent served with afternoon tea. The combination of pineapple and cinnamon is delicious. The smaller, green courgettes are best used for this recipe as they contain less water and more flavour.

120ml rapeseed oil, plus more for the tin
2 small eggs, lightly beaten
150g soft brown sugar
½ tsp vanilla extract
425g can of pineapple rings in fruit juice, drained
2 small courgettes, unpeeled and grated (240g)
225g plain flour
1 tsp bicarbonate of soda
½ tsp baking powder
¾ tsp ground cinnamon
½ tsp sea salt
75g walnuts, finely chopped
120g raisins
15g flaxseed
3 glacé cherries (optional)

1 OF YOUR 5-A-DAY

Preheat the oven to 200°C/fan 180°C/400°F/gas mark 6. Oil a 23 x 13cm loaf tin.

Combine the eggs, oil, sugar and vanilla in a large bowl and blend with a hand-held mixer until thick and foamy. Set aside three rings of pineapple on a piece of kitchen paper to dry. Crush the remaining pineapple and add to the foamy mix with the courgettes.

Sift the flour with the bicarbonate of soda, baking powder, cinnamon and salt, then add to the batter with the nuts, raisins and flaxseed. Blend the mixture well.

Spoon the batter into the prepared tin and bake the loaf for 10 minutes. Working quickly, take the loaf out of the oven briefly and lay the three rings of pineapple on top of the batter, putting one glacé cherry in each ring. (If you add the pineapple rings earlier, they will simply sink into the batter.) Return to the oven as rapidly as possible and bake for a further 50 minutes or until a skewer comes out clean. Leave to cool completely before removing from the tin.

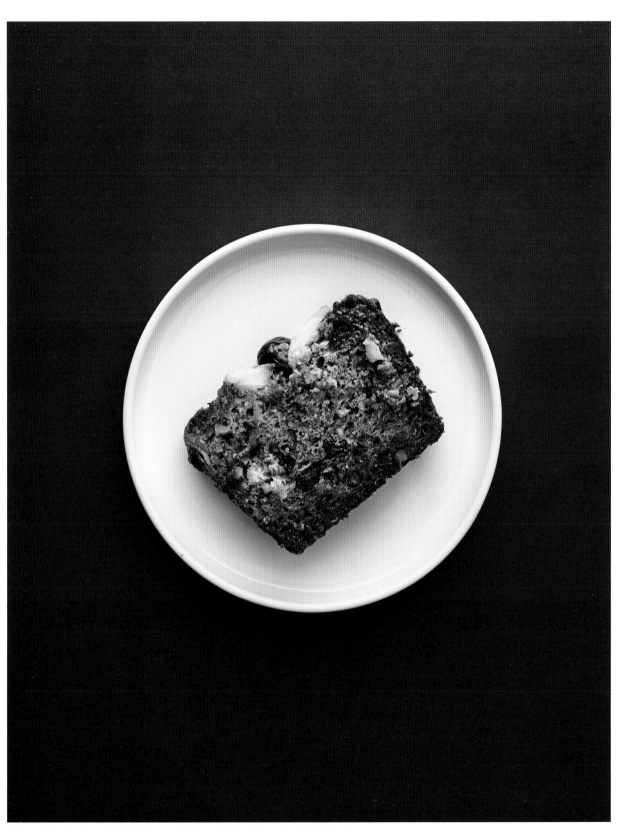

SQUASH AND ORANGE TRAY BAKE | *serves 8*

A light sponge cake perfect for sharing. Very moist with a distinctive orange flavour. If onion squash (also known as red kuri or potimarron) is unavailable or out of season, use butternut squash instead.

For the cake

150g unsalted butter, softened
150g caster sugar
4 eggs
320g onion squash, peeled and
  finely grated
1 tbsp finely grated orange zest
2 oranges, peel and pith removed,
  segmented, then cut into small pieces
60g ripe apricots, cut into small pieces
60g Italian candied mixed orange and
  lemon peel
250g plain flour
1 tsp baking powder
½ tsp bicarbonate of soda

For the topping

30g pumpkin seeds
200g cream cheese
40g icing sugar
1 tbsp finely grated orange zest

1 OF YOUR 5-A-DAY

Preheat the oven to 200°C/fan 180°C/400°F/gas mark 6. Line a 30 x 20cm tray bake tin with baking parchment.

Beat the butter and sugar for five minutes until light in colour. Add the eggs one at a time, mixing well after each addition.

Prepare the squash and oranges and place into a bowl. Drain off and reserve and liquid that is released. Add to the butter mixture with the apricots and mixed candied peel.

Sift the flour with the baking powder and bicarbonate of soda and blend carefully into the wet ingredients. Pour the batter into the prepared tin.

Bake for 35–40 minutes or until it bounces back to the touch. Place on a wire rack, still in the tin, and leave until cool. Turn out of the tin.

For the topping, dry-fry the pumpkin seeds until they pop, then set aside.

Mix the cream cheese with the icing sugar and 2 tbsp of the reserved squash and orange juices and spread on top of the cake. Sprinkle with the pumpkin seeds and orange zest.

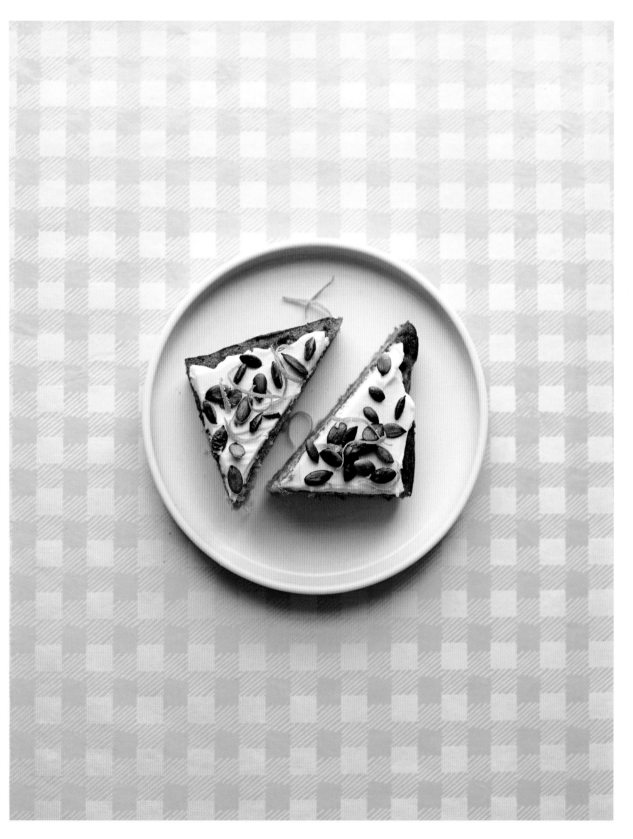

WATERMELON, STRAWBERRY AND MINT CRUSH | *serves 2 (makes 300ml)*

A vibrant red, delicately flavoured and refreshing smoothie. The addition of mint and black pepper provides a tangy finish which lengthens the enjoyment of this drink.

160g watermelon
10 large or 14 small strawberries
6–8 mint leaves, to taste, plus more to serve (optional)
pinch of freshly ground black pepper

2 OF YOUR 5-A-DAY

Remove the pips from the watermelon. Clean the strawberries.

Place everything in a blender, whizz for a minute, then serve with a sprig of mint in each glass, if you like.

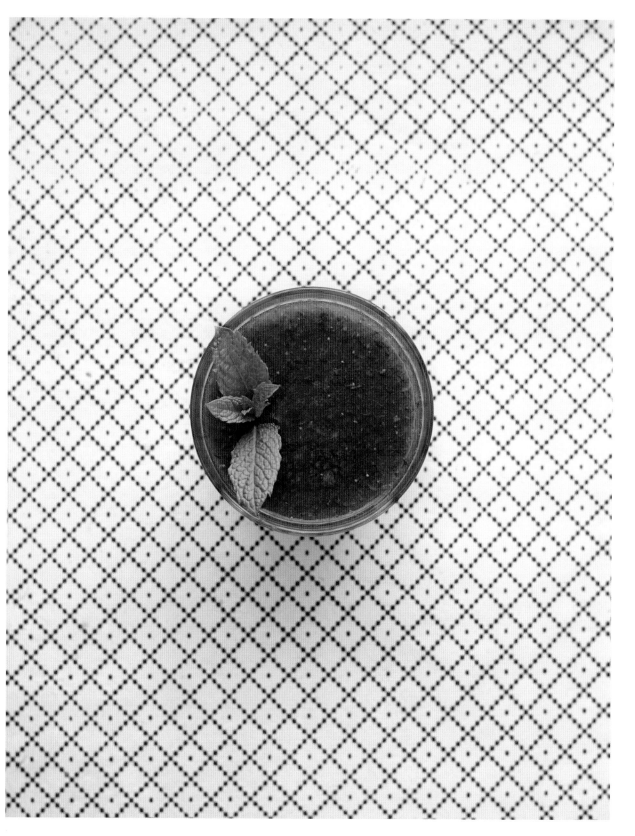

CARROT, APPLE AND GINGER JUICE | *serves 2 (makes 400ml)*

A light flavoursome smoothie with soft tones of raw carrot and ginger. The trick for this smoothie is to blend the apple juice and carrot for a good three or four minutes. This is a great detox drink, with lots of vitamin A.

1 small carrot, finely grated
1 tsp finely chopped root ginger
300ml apple juice
1 ripe pear, such as
   Conference, peeled

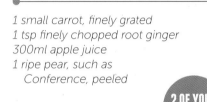

2 OF YOUR 5-A-DAY

Blend the carrot, ginger and apple juice for three to four minutes until smooth. Peel, quarter and core the pear and drop gently into the mix. Blend for one final minute.

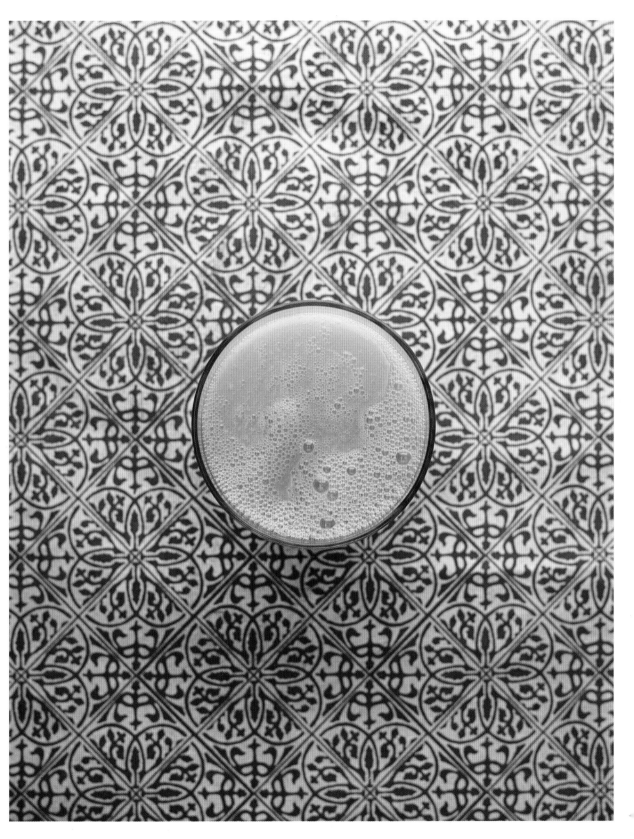

AVOCADO, BANANA AND
RASPBERRY ENERGISER | *serves 2 (makes 350ml)*

A tantalising, thick, restoring smoothie with a lovely rosy colour. The avocado provides plenty of vitamin E as well as a rich velvety texture, and it also balances the sweetness of the banana and raspberry.

handful of raspberries
200ml apple juice, or more for a
   thinner smoothie
½ avocado
1 banana

2 OF YOUR
5-A-DAY

Blend the raspberries with the apple juice. Add the banana and avocado and blend everything together for two minutes.

Adjust the consistency with more apple juice, if needed.

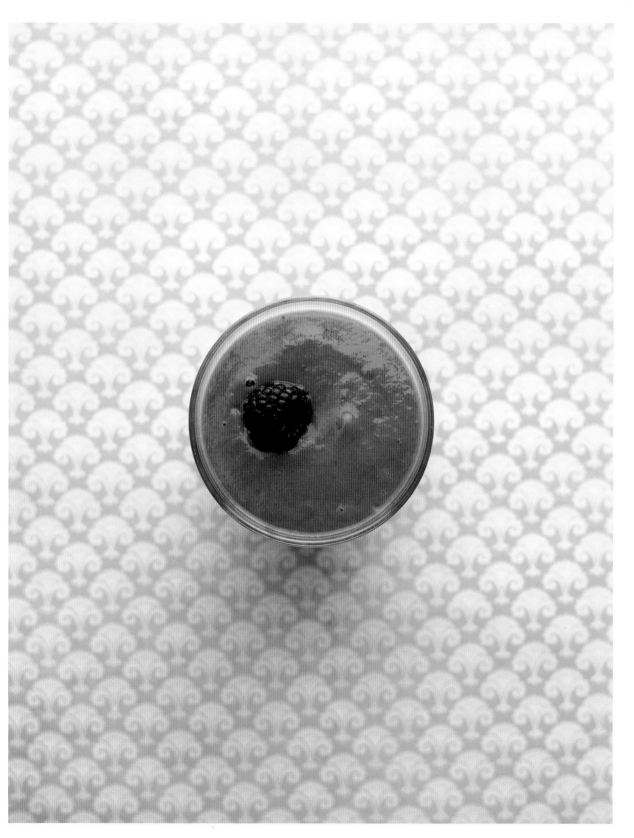

MELON, CUCUMBER AND LIME ZINGER | *serves 2 (makes 320ml)*

The cool, refreshing flavour of the cucumber superbly complements the sweetness of the melon, resulting in an invigorating, light smoothie with a hint of lime.

½ cantaloupe melon, deseeded
½ cucumber
1 lime

2 OF YOUR 5-A-DAY

Scoop out the melon flesh and place in a blender. Add the cucumber and blend for two or three minutes. If the bits are sticking and refusing to break down, switch off the blender, stir briefly, then blend again.

Slice the lime in half, squeeze the juice into a bowl and remove any pips. Add all the juice and any lime flesh to the blender and blend briefly.

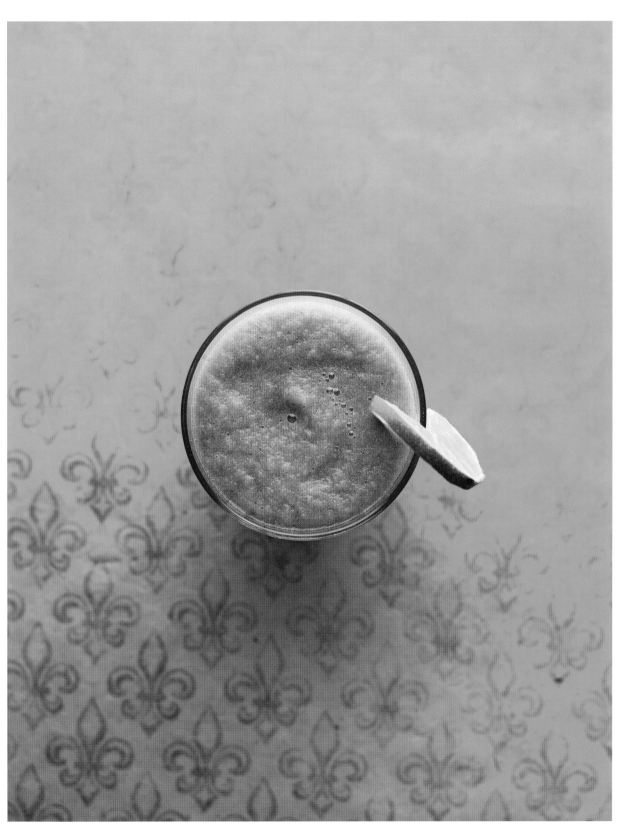

APPLE, BLACKBERRY AND
BEETROOT REFRESHER | *serves 2 (makes 360ml)*

A velvety, airy, deep purple smoothie, full of blood-building beetroot and antioxidant-rich blackberries. A really healthy vitamin-rich drink that tastes delicious.

handful of blackberries
200ml apple juice
½ medium beetroot, peeled and
  finely grated
1 dessert apple, cored and
  finely grated

**2 OF YOUR
5-A-DAY**

Blend the blackberries and the apple juice for two minutes, then strain the juice and discard the blackberry pulp. Place the beetroot and apple into the blender, add the strained juice and blend on high for three or four minutes.

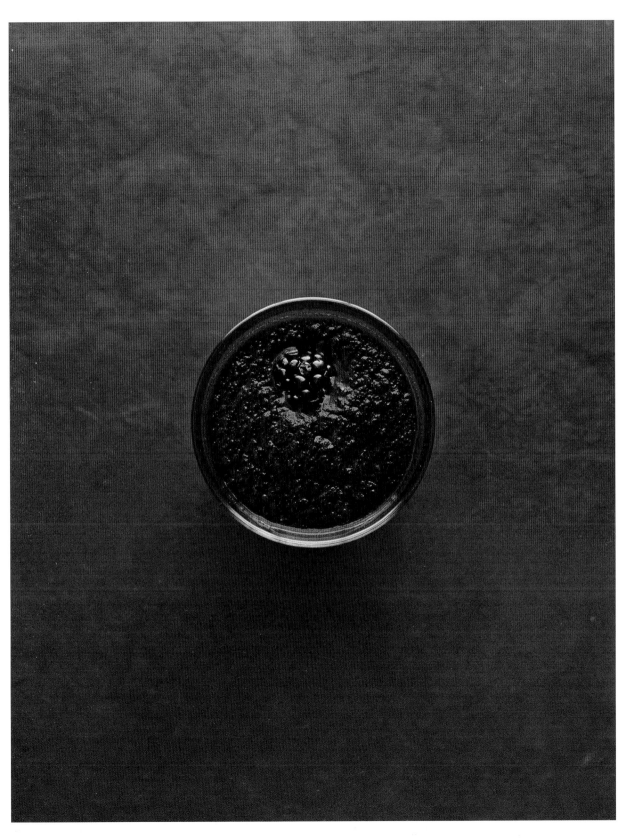

BLOOD ORANGE, PUMPKIN AND FLAXSEED SMOOTHIE | *serves 2 (makes 360ml)*

This breakfast smoothie is enhanced by the addition of flaxseed which is full of omega 3. Substitute the pumpkin with butternut squash if the former is not in season. The lemon adds a tang that will get you going in the morning.

2cm-thick chunk or slice of pumpkin or
    butternut squash (80g)
2 blood oranges
½ lemon
200ml orange juice
1 ripe pear
1 level tbsp flaxseed

2 OF YOUR 5-A-DAY

Peel and finely grate the pumpkin and add to the blender. Squeeze the oranges and lemon into the blender through a sieve and add the extra orange juice.

Peel, quarter and core the pear and add to the blender with the flaxseed. Blend everything for three to five minutes.

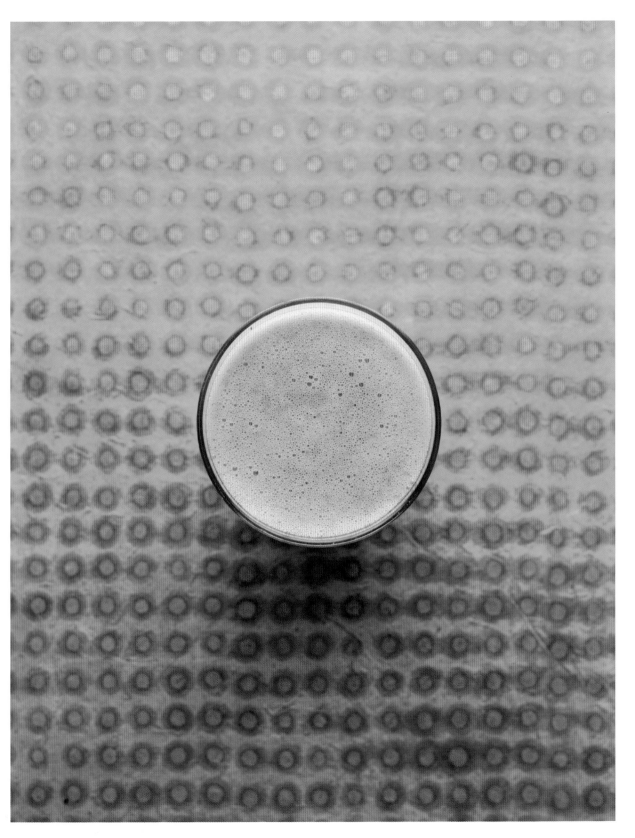

INDEX

THANKS

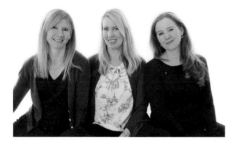

First and foremost we would like to thank Neel Shah, our talented young chef, who perfected many of our recipes at Thrive on Five, and brought us many new ideas for this book. Thanks too to Sarah Main, Lesley Loveday, Susanne Kristensen, Stine Kristensen, Heidi Ali, Senay Harper and Alex Harper for their help in recipe development and for their diligent testing. To Pippa Kershaw for her editing, to Rosie Glenn and Cliff Harden for their creative input, and to Robert Pierce Jones, Liz Straker Grimes and Jussie Burbidge for their general support and guidance as we developed this concept. Many thanks to Anne Furniss and all the team at Quadrille who have shown us their unwavering and dedicated support from day one of this book project. Finally to our families (and tasters!), to Gag and Jules, to Paul, Luke, Fran and Zach, and to Doug, Christian and Anna. They have all shown us great patience as we worked to get Thrive on Five off the ground.

NINA, RANDI AND JO

www.thriveonfive.co.uk

Publishing Director: Anne Furniss
Creative Director: Helen Lewis
Project Editor: Lucy Bannell
Art Direction and Design: Claire Peters
Photography: Dan Jones
Illustration: Shutterstock and Claire Peters
Food consultant: Neel Shah
Food stylist: Lizzie Harris
Props stylist: Rebecca Newport
Production: Vincent Smith, Stephen Lang

First published in 2015 by
Quadrille Publishing Limited
Pentagon House
52–54 Southwark Street
London SE1 1UN

www.quadrille.co.uk

Text © 2015 Nina and Jo Littler and Randi Glenn
Photography © 2015 Dan Jones
Design and layout © 2015 Quadrille Publishing Limited

Cataloguing in Publication Data: a catalogue record for this book is available from the British Library.

ISBN: 978 1 84949 587 5

Printed in China